Fourth Edition

The Development of Language

Jean Berko Gleason
Boston University

Allyn and Bacon

Boston • London • Toronto • Sydney • Tokyo • Singapore

Executive Editor: Stephen D. Dragin
Editorial Assistant: Christine Svitila
Editiorial-Production Administrator: Joe Sweeney
Editorial-Production Service: Walsh & Associates, Inc.
Composition Buyer: Linda Cox
Manufacturing Buyer: Megan Cochran
Cover Administrator: Linda Knowles

Copyright © 1997 by Allyn & Bacon
A Viacom Company
160 Gould Street
Needham Heights, MA 02194
Earlier editions copyright © 1993, 1989 by Macmillan Publishing Company

Internet: www.abacon.com
America Online: keyword: College Online

Library of Congress Cataloging-in-Publication Data
The development of language / [edited by] Jean Berko Gleason. — 4th
   ed.
      p.   cm.
    Includes bibliographical references and indexes.
    ISBN 0-205-19885-6
    1. Language acquisition.   2. Psycholinguistics.
3. Sociolinguistics.   I. Gleason, Jean Berko.
P118.D44 1996
401'.93—dc20   96-27292
                                         CIP

Printed in the United States of America
10 9 8 7 6 5 4 3   00 99 98 97

Photo credits: Robert Harbison, pp. 8, 195, 293, 449; Peter Vandermark/Stock, Boston, p. 101; Deborah Kahn Kalas/Stock, Boston, p. 173; Michael Weisbrot and Family/Stock, Boston, pp. 213, 229; Will Faller, pp. 333, 355, 427; Fredrik D. Bodin/Stock, Boston, pp. 338, 455; Hearing and Speech Clinic, University of Maryland at College Park, p. 371.

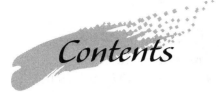

Contents

7 Theoretical Approaches to Language Acquisition 259

John Neil Bohannon III *Butler University*
John D. Bonvillian *University of Virginia*

Introduction 259; Distinguishing Features of Theoretical Approaches
260; Behavioral Approaches 263; Linguistic Approaches 269;
Interactionist Approaches 279; Piaget's Cognitive Approach Information 279;
Processing Approach 284; Social Interaction Approach 290; *Summary and
New Directions 300; Key Words 303; Suggested Projects 303; Suggested
Readings 305; References 306*

8 Individual Differences: Implications for the Study of Language Acquisition 317

Beverly A. Goldfield *Rhode Island College*
Catherine E. Snow *Harvard Graduate School of Education*

Introduction 317; The History of Individual Differences in Child
Language Research 319; Individual Differences in Early Words 321;
Individual Differences in Early Sentences 325; Stability of Individual
Differences 326; Sources of Variation 330; Implications of Individual
Differences for a Theory of Language Acquisition 337; *Summary 340;
Key Words 341; Suggested Projects 341; Suggested Readings 342;
References 342*

9 Atypical Language Development 348

Nan Bernstein Ratner *University of Maryland*

Introduction 348; Communicative Development and Severe Hearing
Impairment 349; Educational Approaches to the Development of
Language in Deaf Children 353; Mental Retardation and Communicative
Development 358; Autism 360; Specific Language Impairment 365;
Atypical Speech Development 375; *Summary 379; Key Words 380;
Suggested Projects 381; Suggested Readings 381; References 383*

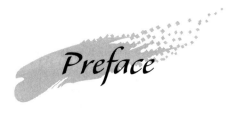

Preface

This is the fourth edition of *The Development of Language,* which is intended for anyone with an interest in how children acquire language and in how language develops over the life span. Each chapter has been written by an expert in a particular area of research, in a way that is accessible to educated nonexperts. This edition has been designed as a text for upper-level undergraduate or graduate courses in language development, or as readings for courses in psycholinguistics, cognitive development, developmental psychology, speech pathology, and related subjects. The book also serves as a resource for professionals in all of the fields just noted.

This edition has been revised extensively to contain state-of-the-art material on all the topics that are covered. The fourth edition also contains new features that we have added in response to suggestions from students, colleagues, and reviewers; these will enhance its value as a text. In particular: (1) major sections have been rewritten to increase their accessibility to readers from diverse backgrounds; (2) language development in the school years has been treated separately from the development of literacy in Chapter 10, with much new information on peers and the media; and (3) a section of Key Words has been added at the end of each chapter. These highlighted words from the chapter also appear in the Glossary, and they provide the reader with a quick way to check the important new terms that have been introduced.

Previous study of linguistics on the part of the reader is not assumed, and each chapter presents its material along with whatever linguistic background information is necessary for understanding. On the other hand, we assume that readers will be familiar with basic concepts in psychology (e.g., *attachment*) and with the work of major figures like Jean Piaget and B. F. Skinner. Most books on language development are concerned only with language acquisition by children, and have tended to assume that development is complete when the most complex syntactic structures have been attained. But linguistic development, like psychological development, is a lifelong process, and so we have set out to illuminate the nature of language development over the life span.

It would be hard for a single author to write this book. The study of language development has grown so rapidly in recent years that there are now many topics that are highly specialized, and it is rare for one person to be an expert in all areas of this expanding field. For instance, there are few investigators who are authorities on the language of both infants and elderly people. Yet both topics are covered here. Fortunately, a number of researchers specializing in major subfields have agreed to contribute to the book; the chapters, therefore, are written by authors who not only know their topic well, but are known for their research in it. They present what they consider to be the salient ideas and the most recent and relevant studies in their own areas.

Since development is always the result of an interaction between innate capacities and environmental forces, we take an interactive perspective, one that takes into account both the biological endowment that makes language possible and the environmental factors that foster development. Our theoretical perspective has remained the same—both interactive and eclectic—but we have tried to add new material that represents the field, even if it does not necessarily represent our own views. Theory remains a controversial area in psycholinguistics; the most important theoretical positions are presented here, along with their strengths and weaknesses, in what we hope is an evenhanded but thought-provoking approach. We count proponents of each of the divergent theories among our personal friends, and value their continued friendship.

We have had to be selective in our choice of major topics, and some of our favorite subjects have, of necessity, been omitted. There are so many different topics that are now recognized in the study of language development that it is impossible to include them all in one cohesive book. And we have not attempted to include cross-cultural and bilingual studies that rely on knowledge of languages other than English.

We also have a newly revised instructor's manual and test bank prepared by Pam Gleason, available to instructors who use the book as a text. The manual provides helpful outlines of the chapters, emphasizes key points, and provides suggestions for classroom activities. A number of the authors here can be seen in the Public Broadcasting Service NOVA production on language development called "Babytalk," which is still available in some areas; more recently, PBS has made available a videotaped college course called "Discovering Psychology," with a half-hour program (#6) devoted to early language development.

It is impossible to edit a book without becoming indebted to many people; I am grateful, first of all, to the authors who agreed to contribute to this volume, and I welcome John Bonvillian and Richard Ely, who are new contributors. Thanks also to Kris Farnsworth and Stephen Dragin, our editors at Allyn & Bacon, and to Mary Perry at Boston University, who, as ever, has been immensely helpful in every way. I thank the following reviewers for their comments and suggestions: Martin Fujiki, Brigham Young University; and Elda Buchanan, Bradley University.

My family is due thanks as well: My husband, Andrew Gleason, for his patience, and my daughters Katherine, Pam, and Cynthia, now grown, whose developing language was a source of inspiration and joy. Some of their early pronouncements, like "My teacher holded the baby rabbits and we patted them," have been quoted so often they should be in *Bartlett's*.

—Jean Berko Gleason

Chapter One

The Development of Language: An Overview and a Preview

Jean Berko Gleason, *Boston University*

Introduction

Why do we study language development? This phenomenal yet basically universal human achievement poses some of the most challenging theoretical and practical questions of our times: How and why do young children acquire complex grammar? What if no one spoke to them—would children invent language by themselves? Are humans unique, or can language be taught to higher primates? Are there theories or models that can adequately account for language development? Is language a separate capacity, or is it simply one facet of our general cognitive ability? What is it that individuals actually must know in order to have full adult competence in language, and to what extent is the development of those skills representative of universal processes? What about individual differences? What happens when language develops atypically, and is there anything we can do about it? What happens to language skills as one grows older—what is acquired, and what is lost? These are some of the questions that intrigue language-development researchers, and they have led to the plan of this book.

Children in every part of the world, regardless of the degree of grammatical or phonological complexity, acquire the major components of their native language by the time they are three or four years old. By the time they are of school age and begin the formal study of grammar, they already can vary their speech to suit the social and communicative nature of a situation, they know the meaning and pronunciation of literally thousands of words, and they use quite correctly the grammatical forms—subjects, objects, verbs, plurals, and tenses—whose names they learn only in the late elementary years. Language development, however, does not cease when the individual reaches school age or, for that matter, adolescence or maturity—the developmental process continues throughout the life cycle. The reorganization and reintegration of mental processes that are typical of other intellectual functions can also be seen in language, as the changing conditions that accompany maturity lead to modification of linguistic capacity. This book, therefore, is written from a developmental perspective that encompasses the life span. Since most studies of language development have centered on children, this preponderance is reflected in the research reported here. The major questions addressed, however, are not limited to what can be learned from the study of children and, in fact, require the study of mature individuals as well.

This chapter is divided into four major sections:

The first section provides a brief overview of *the course of language development* from early infancy to old age. It contains a preview of the chapters that follow (the major topics included are treated at length in later chapters of the book).

The second section notes some of the unique *biological foundations* for language that make its development possible in humans. Biological factors are necessary, but they are not sufficient to ensure language development, which does not occur without social interaction.

The third section describes the major *linguistic systems* that individuals must acquire. No particular linguistic theory is espoused here; instead, descriptive techniques are used that have provided the framework for much basic research in language acquisition, and more technical linguistic material is presented in the appropriate substantive chapter. If there is a unifying perspective that the authors of this book share, it is the view that individuals acquire during their lives an **internalized representation** of language that is systematic in nature and amenable to study. This does not imply that inner representation could be established in the absence of social contact, or without several different types of learning (as Chapter 7 on theoretical perspectives makes clear).

The fourth and final section of this chapter focuses on the background and methods of the *study of language development.*

An Overview of the Course of Language Development

Communication Development in Infancy

During their first months, human beings begin to acquire the communicative skills that underlie language, long before they say their first words. Babies are intensely social beings; they gaze into the eyes of their caregivers and are sensitive to the emotional tone of the voices around them. They pay attention to the language spoken to them; they take their turn in conversation, even if that turn is only a burble (Masataka, 1993; Snow, 1977). If they want something, they learn to make their intentions known. In addition to possessing the social motivations that are evidenced so early in life, data now show that infants are also physiologically equipped to process incoming speech signals; they are even capable of making fine distinctions among speech sounds that are both rare in the world's languages and previously unknown to them (Eimas, 1975; Werker & Tees, 1984). The latest evidence available suggests that by the age of six months babies have already begun to categorize the sounds of their own language, much as adult speakers do (Kuhl, Williams, Lacerda, Stevens, & Lindblom, 1992).

Midway through their first year, infants begin to babble, playing with sound much as they play with their fingers and toes. There is considerable controversy over the relation between babbling and talking (Blake & Boysson-Bardies, 1992; Boysson-Bardies & Vihman, 1991; Jakobson, 1968); however, most researchers now believe that babbling blends into early speech and may continue even after the appearance of recognizable words. At approximately the same age that they take their first steps, many infants produce their first words. Like walking, early language appears at around the same age and in much the same way all over the world, regardless of the degree of sophistication of the society. The relative ease of pronunciation of a language and its degree of grammatical complexity do not appear to affect the age at which children begin to speak (Lenneberg, 1967). The early precursors of language that arise during the first year of life are discussed in Chapter 2.

Phonological Development: Learning Sounds and Sound Patterns

Once infants have begun to speak, the course of language development appears to have some universal characteristics (Brown, 1973). Typically, toddlers' early utterances are only one word long, and the words are simple in pronunciation and concrete in meaning (Stoel-Gammon & Cooper, 1984). They refer to the objects, events, and people in the child's immediate surroundings—words like *hi, doggie, mommy,* and *juice* (Bloom, 1970; Clark, 1993; Nelson & Lucariello, 1985). Here, as in other areas of linguistic research, it is important to recognize that different constraints act upon the child's **comprehension** and **production** of a particular form. Some sounds are more difficult to pronounce than others, and combinations of consonants may prove particularly problematic. Within a given language, children solve the phonological problems they encounter in varying ways. A framework for the study of children's growing ability to both recognize and produce the sounds of their language is provided in Chapter 3.

Semantic Development: Learning the Meanings of Words

The ways in which speakers relate words to their referents and their meanings are the subject matter of **semantic development**. Just as there are constraints on the phonological shapes of children's early words, there appear to be limits on the kinds of meanings that those early words embody—for instance, very young children are more likely to have in their vocabularies words that refer to objects that move *(bus)* than objects that are immobile *(bench)*. Their vocabularies reflect their daily lives, and are unlikely to refer to events that are distant in time or space or to anything of an abstract nature. As they enter the school years, children's words become increasingly complex and interconnected, and children also gain a new kind of knowledge: **metalinguistic awareness.** This new ability makes it possible for them to think about their language, understand what words are, and even define them (Papandropoulou & Sinclair, 1974; Snow, 1990). Investigations of children's first words and their meanings, as well as the ways in which early meaning systems become elaborated into complex semantic networks, are discussed in Chapter 4.

Putting Words Together: Morphology and Syntax in the Preschool Years

Sometime during their second year, after they know about fifty words, most children progress to a stage of two-word combinations (Brown, 1973). Words that they said in the one-word stage are now combined into these **telegraphic** utterances, without articles, prepositions, inflections, or any of the other grammatical modifications that adult language requires. The child can now say such things as "That doggie," meaning "That is a doggie," and "Mommy juice," meaning "Mommy's juice" or "Mommy, give me my juice" or "Mommy is drinking her juice."

An examination of children's two-word utterances in many different language communities (Brown, 1973; Slobin, 1979) has shown that everywhere in the world children at this age are expressing the same kinds of thoughts and intentions in the same kinds of utterances. They ask for more of something; they say no to something; they notice something, or they notice that it has disappeared. This leads them to produce utterances like "More milk!" "No bed!" "Hi, kitty!" and "All-gone cookie!"

A little later in the two-word stage, another dozen or so kinds of meanings appear. For instance, children may name an actor and a verb: "Daddy eat." They modify a noun: "Bad doggie." They specify a location: "Kitty table." They name a verb and an object, leaving out the subject: "Eat lunch." At this stage, children are expressing these basic meanings but they cannot use the language forms that indicate number, gender, and tense. Even in a highly inflected language (such as Hebrew) in which it would be impossible to speak the root word without some of these markers, children settle on one form, which they use indiscriminately: Girls, for example, frequently use the feminine form of words, regardless of the grammatical requirements (Dromi & Berman, 1982). Toddler language is in the here and now; there is no tomorrow and no yesterday in language at the two-word stage. What children can say is closely related to their level of cognitive and social development, and a child who cannot conceive of the past is unlikely to speak of it. As the child's utterances grow longer, grammatical forms begin to appear. In English, articles, prepositions, and inflections representing number, person, and tense begin to be heard. Although the two-word stage has some universal characteristics across all languages, what is acquired next depends on the features of the language being learned. English-speaking children learn the articles *a* and *the*, but in a language such as Russian there are no articles. Russian grammar, on the other hand, has features that English grammar does not. One remarkable finding has been that children acquiring a given language do so in essentially the same order. In English, for instance, children learn *in* and *on* before other prepositions such as *under*. After they learn regular plurals and pasts, like *nooses* and *heated,* they create some **overregularized** forms of their own, like *gooses* and *eated.*

Researchers account for children's early utterances in varying ways, however. The work of the 1960s, inspired by grammatical theory (Chomsky, 1957, 1965), interpreted early word combinations as evidence that the child was a young crypto-grapher, endowed with a cognitive impetus to develop syntax and a grammatical system. More recently, the child's intentions and need to communicate them to others have been looked to for explanations of grammatical development. But children's unique ability to acquire complex grammar, regardless of the motivation behind it, remains at the heart of linguistic inquiry. The learning of morphological systems, such as the plural or past tense (Berko, 1958), remains some of the strongest evidence we have that children are not simply learning bits and pieces of the adult linguistic system but are constructing generative systems of their own. Early sentences and the acquisition of morphology are examined in Chapter 5.

Language in Social Contexts

Language development includes acquiring the necessary ability to use language appropriately in a multiplicity of social situations. The system of rules that dictates the way language is used to accomplish social ends is called **pragmatics.** An individual who acquires the phonology, morphology, syntax, and semantics of a language has acquired **linguistic competence.** A sentence such as "Excuse me, but might I borrow your pencil for a moment?" certainly shows that the speaker has linguistic competence, since it is obviously perfectly grammatical. If, however, this sentence is addressed to a two-year-old, it is just as certainly inappropriate; more appropriate would be something like "Give me the pencil—that's right, give it to me." Linguistic competence is not sufficient; speakers must also acquire **communicative competence** (Hymes, 1972), or the ability to vary their language appropriately in a variety of situations; in other words, it requires knowledge of pragmatics. During the preschool years, young children learn to express a variety of **speech acts,** such as polite requests, or clarification of their own utterances. Their parents are particularly eager that they learn to be polite (Snow, Perlmann, Gleason, & Hooshyar, 1990). Speakers ultimately learn important variations in language that serve to mark their gender, regional origin, social class, and occupation. Other necessary variations are associated with such things as the social setting, topic of discourse, and characteristics of the person being addressed. The use of language in social contexts is discussed in Chapter 6.

Theoretical Approaches to Language Acquisition

In general, explaining what it is that children acquire during the course of language development is easier than explaining how they do it. Do parents shape their children's early babbling into speech through reinforcement and teaching strategies? Or is language, perhaps, an independent and **innate** faculty, built into the human biobehavioral system? Learning theorists and linguistic theorists do not agree on these basic principles. Between the theoretical poles represented by learning theorists on the one hand and linguistic theorists on the other, lie three different interactionist perspectives: (1) *Cognitive developmentalists* believe that language is just one facet of human cognition, and that children in acquiring language are basically learning to put words to concepts they have already acquired. (2) *Information theorists* who study language are also interested in human cognition, but from the perspective of the neural architecture that supports it. They see children as processors of information, and they use the computer to model the ways neural connections supporting language are strengthened through exposure to adult speech. (3) *Social interactionist theorists* emphasize the child's motivation to communicate with others. They emphasize the role that the special features of **child-directed speech (CDS)** may play in facilitating children's language acquisition. A discussion and an evaluation of the theories that have been put forth to explain language development are included in Chapter 7.

Individual Differences: Implications for the Study of Language Acquisition

Even though this brief overview has emphasized the regularities and continuities that have been observed in the development of language, it is important to know that individual differences have been found in almost every aspect, even during the earliest period of development. In the acquisition of phonology, for instance, some children are quite conservative and avoid words they have difficulty pronouncing; others are willing to take a chance. Early words and early word combinations reveal different strategies in acquiring language. Although much of linguistic inquiry has been directed at finding commonalities across children in language acquisition, it is important to remember that there is also variation in the onset of speech, the rate at which language develops, and the style of language used by the child. This should not surprise us, since we know that babies differ in temperament, cognitive style, and in many other ways; variation is a very healthy part of our genetic heritage. In addition, children's early language may reflect the preferences of adults in a society—for instance, American parents stress the names of things, but nouns might not be so important in all societies. Individual differences must be accounted for by any comprehensive theory of language development, and they must be taken into account by those who work with children. Individual differences are the topic of Chapter 8.

Atypical Language Development

Language has been a human endowment for so many millenia that it is exceptionally robust; as we shall see, it is under most circumstances almost impossible to suppress. There are conditions, however, that may lead to atypical language development—for instance, sensory problems such as deafness. In this case the capacity for language is intact, but lack of accessible auditory input makes the acquisition of oral language difficult; children with hearing impairments who learn a manual language such as **American Sign Language** (ASL), however, are able to communicate in a complete and sophisticated language.

Children who are diagnosed as mentally retarded, such as most children with **Down syndrome,** may show rather typical patterns of language development, but at a slower rate than normally developing children. Children with **autism** frequently exhibit patterns of language development that are atypical in multiple ways; they may have particular problems, for instance, using language that deals with the emotional states of others (Tager-Flusberg & Sullivan, 1995). Occasionally children suffer from **specific language impairment,** problems in language development accompanied by no other obvious physical, sensory, or emotional difficulties. Still other children have particular problems producing speech, even though their internal representation of language is intact: They may stutter or have motor impairments. Atypical language development, and its relation to the processes described in earlier chapters, is the subject of Chapter 9.

Language and Literacy in the School Years

By the time they get to kindergarten, children have amassed a vocabulary of about 8,000 words and almost all of the basic grammatical forms of their language. They can handle questions, negative statements, dependent clauses, compound sentences, and a great variety of other constructions. They have also learned much more than vocabulary and grammar—they have learned to use language in many different social situations. They can, for instance, talk baby talk to babies, be rude to their friends, and act somewhat polite with their grandparents. Their communicative competence is growing.

During the school years, children are increasingly called upon to interact with peers; peer speech is quite different from speech to parents, and it is often both

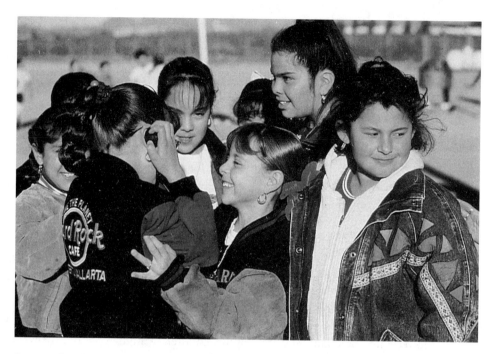

During the school years children acquire new linguistic skills as they interact with peers. Explaining how to build a fire or telling a joke requires connected discourse and decontextualized language.

humorous and aggressive. Jokes, riddles, and play with language constitute a substantial portion of their spontaneous speech. Faced with many new models, school-aged children also learn from television and films, and their speech may be marked by expressions from their favorite entertainments.

New cognitive attainments in the school years make it possible for children to talk in ways that they could not as preschoolers, and to think about language itself—they may even have favorite words (like *pumpernickel*) that are not necessarily their favorite things. They become increasingly adept at producing connected, multi-utterance speech and can now produce narratives that describe their past experience. In order to succeed in school, children must also learn to use **decontextualized language**—language that is not tied to the here and now. In addition to their narrative skills, they now develop the ability to provide explanations and descriptions using decontextualized language (Snow, 1983).

The attainment of literacy marks a major milestone in children's development, and it calls upon both their metalinguistic abilities (for instance, they must understand what a word is), and their new abilities to use decontextualized language. Study of the cognitive processes involved in reading and the development of adequate models that represent the acquisition of this skill are two topics that actively involve researchers in developmental psycholinguistics.

Children who come from literate households know a great deal about reading and writing before formal instruction begins, and thus are at an advantage in school. Once children have acquired the ability to read and write, these new skills, in turn, have profound effects upon their spoken language. Learning to read is not an easy task for all children; this extremely complex activity requires intricate coordination of a number of separate abilities. Humans have been speaking since the earliest days of our prehistory, but reading has been a common requirement only in very modern times; we should not be surprised, therefore, that reading skills vary greatly in the population. Reading problems as exemplified in the **dyslexias** pose serious theoretical and practical problems for the psycholinguistic researcher. The acquisition of language and the development of literacy skills during the school years and through adolescence are discussed in Chapter 10.

Development and Loss: Changes in the Adult Years

In the normal course of events, language development, like cognitive development, moral development, or psychological development, continues beyond the point where the individual has assumed the outward appearance of an adult. During the teen years, young people acquire their own special style, and part of being a successful teenager rests in knowing how to talk like one. Now, in adulthood, there are new linguistic attainments.

Language is involved in psychological development; the psychiatrist Erik Erikson (1959) pointed out that one of the major life tasks facing young people is the formation of an identity, a sense of who they are. A distinct personal linguistic style is part of one's special identity. Further psychological goals of early adulthood that call for expanded linguistic skills include beginning an occupation and establishing intimate relations with others.

Language development during the adult years varies greatly among individuals, depending on such things as level of education and social and occupational roles. Actors, for instance, must learn not only to be heard by large audiences but to speak the words of others using varying voices and regional dialects. Working people learn the special tones of voice and terminology associated with their own occupational register or code.

With advancing age, numerous linguistic changes take place. For instance, some word-finding difficulty is inevitable—the inability to produce a name that is "on the tip of the tongue" is a phenomenon that becomes increasingly familiar as one approaches retirement age. Hearing loss and impairments of memory can affect an older person's ability to communicate. But not all changes are for the worse—vocabulary increases, as does narrative skill. In preliterate societies, for instance, the official storytellers are typically older members of the community. Although most individuals remain linguistically vigorous in their later years, language deterioration becomes severe for some, and they may lose both comprehension and voluntary speech. The aphasias and dementias exact their linguistic toll on affected individuals, whose speech may become as limited as that of young children. Language development in adulthood and the later years is described in Chapter 11.

The Biological Bases of Language

Animal Communication Systems

Human language has special properties that have led many researchers to conclude that such language is both **species specific** and **species uniform**; that is, it is unique to humans and essentially similar in all humans (Lenneberg, 1967; Marler, 1990). The characteristics that distinguish human language are illuminated when they are compared with those of animal communication systems. Animals are clearly able to communicate at some level with one another as well as with humans. Cats and dogs meow and bark for attention and are able to convey a variety of messages by methods such as scratching at the door or looking expectantly at their dishes. Scratching, meowing, and gazing hopefully are clearly not language, however; the messages are very limited in scope and can be interpreted only in the context of the immediate situation.

Bee Communication

Insects such as bees have been shown to have an elaborate communication system. Ethologist Karl von Frisch (1950) began to study bees in the 1920s and won a Nobel Prize in 1973 for his studies of communication among these highly social insects. Unlike the expressive meowing of a hungry cat, in many senses the communication system of the bee is referential—it tells other bees about something in the outside world. A bee returning to the hive after finding nectar-filled flowers collects an audience and then performs a dance that indicates the direction and the approximate distance of the nectar from the hive. Other bees watch, join the dance, and then head for the flowers. The bee's dance is actually a miniature form of the trip to the flowers, rather than a symbolic statement. There is nothing symbolic or arbitrary about dancing toward the north to indicate that other bees should fly in that direction. Moreover, although the movements of the dance have structure and meaning, there is only one possible conversational topic—where to find nectar. Even this repertoire is seriously limited; bees cannot, for instance, tell one another that the flowers are pretty or that they just hate gathering nectar.

Sea Mammals and Birds

Many animals have ways of communicating with other members of their species. Whales and dolphins employ elaborate systems of whistles and grunts that are clearly meaningful to other whales and dolphins (Herman, 1981; Savage-Rumbaugh, 1993). Some birds have been shown to have a variety of meaningful calls. Jackdaws, for instance, were studied by Konrad Lorenz (1971), who shared von Frisch's Nobel Prize. Lorenz showed that these relatives of the crow have courting calls, a call for flying away, and one for flying home. They also have a warning rattle that they sound before attacking any other creature carrying a dangling black object. (He discovered this while carrying [dangling] his black swimsuit!)

All of these communication systems have clear utility for the animals that use them, and each one resembles human language in some respect, but they are all tied to the stimulus situation, limited to the here and now and to a restricted set of messages. Human language has characteristics not found in their entirety in these other systems.

Researchers concerned with criteria for what constitutes *language* have produced lists of characteristics that vary somewhat in both length and scope. Most would agree, however, on at least these three cited by Roger Brown (1973):

1. True language is marked by *productivity* in the sense that speakers can make many new utterances and can recombine the forms they already know to say things they have never before heard.

2. It also has *semanticity;* that is, it can represent ideas, events, and objects symbolically.

3. It offers the possibility of *displacement*—messages need not be tied to the immediate context.

Human language enables its users to comment on any aspect of their experience and to consider the past and the future, as well as referents that may be continents away or only in the imagination. The natural communication systems of bees and lower animals do not meet these criteria of language.

Recent attempts to teach language to talking birds, however, have produced some extremely provocative results. For instance, an African grey parrot named Alex has been trained to recognize objects, colors, and shapes and to answer questions about them in English. Faced with an array of things, he is asked, "What object is green?" Alex says, correctly, "wood." He is right about 80 percent of the time (Pepperberg, 1991). More recent experiments with young grey parrots have shown that they can learn to label common objects if they have human tutors who provide interactive lessons; they do not learn from passive listening to lessons on audiotape or from watching videotapes, but do best when the words are presented in context by a friendly and informative person (Pepperberg, 1994). Do African grey parrots have the same sort of linguistic skill human children do? One view is that they do not, and that the birds are responding to complex learned cues. Another interpretation of the evidence is that language is a continuum on which grey parrots have clearly alighted. These parrots are all relatively young (Alex's twentieth birthday is in 1996), and they have a life span of as much as eighty years, so we can afford to reserve judgment on these remarkable birds.

Primate Language

During the past half-century, a great deal of curiosity has focused on the possibility that the higher primates might be capable of learning human language. Chimpanzees are intelligent, social, and communicative animals (Maple & Cone, 1981; Miles, 1983). They use a variety of vocal cries in their life in the wild, including a food bark and a danger cry. Chimpanzees possess genetic structures very similar to our own and are our closest relatives in the animal world (Diamond, 1992). There have been numerous attempts to teach language to chimpanzees and at least one major gorilla language project (Bonvillian & Patterson, 1993; Patterson & Cohn, 1990). The ape studies have provided us with much useful and controversial data on the ability of nonhumans to acquire our language forms. Some of these studies, such as those of David and Ann James Premack (1976), have taught chimpanzees to manipulate artificial symbols (colored plastic tokens) in order to communicate with humans. In another study, researchers taught chimpanzees to use a computer console to send messages (Rumbaugh, 1977). We will concentrate here on some studies that have set out to teach natural language to chimpanzees.

Gua and Viki. In 1931, Professor and Mrs. W. N. Kellogg became the first American family to raise a chimpanzee and a child together (Kellogg, 1980). The Kelloggs brought into their home Gua, a seven-month-old chimpanzee, who stayed with them and their infant son Donald for nine months. No special effort was made to teach Gua to talk; like the human baby, she was simply exposed to a speaking household. During this period, Gua came to use some of her natural chimpanzee cries rather consistently; for instance, she used her food bark not just for food but for anything at all that she wanted. Although Gua was rather better than Donald in most physical accomplishments, unlike Donald she did not babble and did not learn to say any English words.

In the 1940s, psychologists Catherine and Keith Hayes (Hayes, 1951) set out to improve upon the Kelloggs' experiment by raising a chimpanzee named Viki as if she were their own child. They took her home when she was six weeks old, and she remained with them for several years. The Hayeses made every effort to teach Viki to talk; they had assumed that chimpanzees were rather like institutionalized retarded children, and that love and patient instruction would afford Viki the opportunity for optimal language development. After six years of training, Viki appeared to understand a great deal, but she was able to produce, with great difficulty, only four words:

mama, papa, cup, and *up.* She was never able to say more, and in order to pronounce a /p/, she had to hold her lips together with her fingers. Since speech is an **overlaid function,** that is, the organs involved in its production (such as the tongue and lungs) all have primary functions other than language, it requires an extraordinary degree of physiological coordination to articulate while continuing with functions such as breathing and swallowing. From the Hayeses' research it became clear that chimpanzees do not have the specialized articulatory and physiological abilities that make spoken language possible.

In more recent times, other researchers have concluded that the inability to speak may not preclude the possibility of having language. The deaf community in the United States, for instance, uses a gestural rather than a spoken language, American Sign Language (ASL). ASL is a complete language, with its own elaborated grammar and a rich vocabulary, all of which can be conveyed by the shape and movement of the hands in front of the body; it is the equal of vocal language in its capacity to communicate complex human thought (Fischer, 1993; Klima & Bellugi, 1979). A new appreciation of the richness of ASL led to innovative experiments with chimpanzees.

Washoe. The first attempt to capitalize on the ability to comprehend language and the natural gestural ability of a chimpanzee by teaching her signed human language (ASL) was made by Drs. Beatrice and Allen Gardner at the University of Nevada in 1966 (Gardner & Gardner, 1969). The Gardners moved a young chimpanzee named Washoe into a trailer behind their house and began to teach her ASL. Washoe was ten months old at the time and had been captured in the wild in Africa. During the time she was involved in this project, she learned over 130 ASL signs, as well as how to combine them into utterances of several signs (Gardner & Gardner, 1980; see also 1984a, 1984b). On seeing her trainer, she was able to sign, "Please tickle hug hurry," "Gimme food drink," and similar requests.

Washoe was able to sign many of the same things that are found in the language of children in the very early stages of language acquisition, before they learn the grammatical refinements of their own language (Brown, 1970; Van Cantfort & Rimpau, 1982). She appeared to use her signs in a creative way: on seeing a duck for the first time, she signed "water bird." Since her utterances were typically answers to questions posed to her (e.g., "What is that?"), it is not clear whether she was attempting to make a new word, or simply saying that it was water *and* a bird. Unlike English-speaking children, she did not pay attention to word order, and at the time her training ceased in the fifty-first month, it was not clear if her sign language was actually grammatically structured in the sense that even a young child's is (Brown, 1970: Klima & Bellugi, 1972). However, through vocabulary tests of Washoe, as well as of subsequent chimpanzee subjects, the Gardners were able to demonstrate that children's and chimpanzees' first fifty words are very similar.

Moreover, the chimpanzees extended or generalized their words in much the same way that humans do—for instance, once they knew the ASL sign, calling a hat they had never seen before *hat* (Gardner & Gardner, 1984a; 1984b). The question of whether a chimpanzee was capable of syntax remained open. This is an important theoretical question, because syntax makes *productivity*, one of the hallmarks of human language, possible. On the practical side, the remarkable successes attained with chimps have led to innovative programs that teach sign language to communicatively handicapped children.

Nim Chimpsky. An attempt to answer the question of whether chimpanzees can make grammatical sentences was made by Columbia University professor Herbert S. Terrace (1980). Terrace adopted a young male chimp, whom he named Nim Chimpsky. The plan was to raise Nim in a rich human environment, teach him ASL, and then analyze the chimp's emerging ability to combine signs into utterances, paying special attention to any evidence that he could indeed produce grammatical signed sentences. Nim began to sign early: He produced his first sign, "drink," when he was only four months old. But his later utterances never progressed much beyond the two- or three-sign stage. He signed, "Eat Nim," and, "Banana me eat," but when he made four-sign utterances, he added no new information and, unlike even young children, he used no particular word order. He signed, "Banana me eat banana," in which the additional word is merely repetitive. Analyzing the extensive data collected in this project, Terrace concluded that there was no evidence that the chimp could produce anything that might be called a sentence.

An even more serious question regarding the chimpanzee's linguistic capability was raised after Terrace and his associates studied the videotaped interactions of young Nim and his many teachers. They found that Nim understood little about conversational turn-taking, often interrupting his teachers, and that very little of what Nim signed actually originated with the chimp. Most of what he signed was prompted by the teacher and contained major constituents of the teacher's signed utterance to him.

Terrace carried his study further by analyzing films made available to him by other ape-language projects and arrived at the same conclusion: Much of what the chimps signed had just been signed to them. The signing chimps appeared to be responding at least in part to subtle cues from their trainers. The question of the apes' potential was not completely settled by this study, since Terrace himself was aware of the inevitable shortcomings in his project. As Nim reached maturity, he became difficult to work with and was eventually retired to Black Beauty Ranch in Texas, a guest of the Fund for Animals (Vittorini, 1991).

Kanzi. Although it may be true that apes are not capable of language as we know it, the chimpanzee studies have indicated that there are substantial similarities between very young children's and chimpanzees' abilities to engage in symbolic communication (Greenfield & Savage-Rumbaugh, 1991).

Current research by D. M. Rumbaugh and E. S. Savage-Rumbaugh with a pygmy chimp named Kanzi at the Yerkes Center in Atlanta (Savage-Rumbaugh,

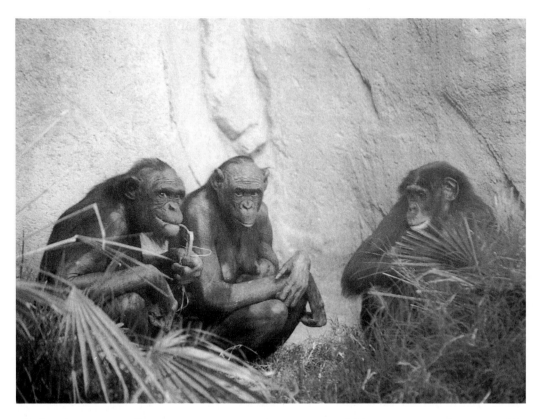

The bonobo, or pygmy chimpanzee, possesses a genetic stucture much like our own. Bonobos are sociable, interactive, and have shown remarkable abilities to communicate. Photo courtesy Roberta Gallagher ©.

1990; Savage-Rumbaugh & Lewin, 1994) has given rise to new hope and speculation about primate linguistic ability. Prior chimpanzee studies used the common chimp *(pan troglodytes)*. The pygmy chimpanzee or bonobo *(p. paniscus)* was virtually unheard of until the mid-1970s.

Pygmy chimpanzees are found only in the remote rain forests of Zaire. They are smaller, less aggressive, more social, more intelligent, and more communicative than the common chimp. Kanzi surprised his trainers when he acquired some manual signs merely by observing his mother's lessons. He is currently the subject of an intensive longitudinal study.

Kanzi has a large, free area in which to roam, and many opportunities to learn both spoken and signed language, as well as how to make tools and carry out everyday activities like cooking dinner. He is now fifteen years old (in 1996) and weighs around 130 pounds. Although he is sexually mature (and they hope he will get to be a father), the Rumbaughs believe they will be able to continue working with him. Studies of his understanding of spoken English show that he comprehends many unusual utterances and can carry out the acts described in them with remarkable accuracy. For instance, if asked to "put the mushroom in the potty," Kanzi obligingly does so, proving that he is attending to language, and not simply carrying out activities that are evident from the nonverbal situation. Current work with Kanzi has led his trainers to be very optimistic about the chimp's progress. Whether the pygmy chimpanzee is the hope of the future in animal language studies remains to be seen.

The Biological Base: Humans

Language in humans is clearly dependent on their having a society in which to learn it, other humans to speak to, and the emotional motivation and intelligence to make it possible; humans also appear to have evolved with specialized neural mechanisms that subserve language. Human beings who are physiologically and psychologically intact will acquire the language of those around them if they grow up among people who speak to them (Locke, 1990). This human interaction seems necessary; there is no evidence that infants can acquire language from watching television, for instance. There are some strong arguments for the case that human language is biologically determined—that it owes its existence to specialized structures in the brain and in the neurological systems of humans. Some of these biological specifications underlie the social and affective characteristics of infants that tie them to the adults around them and serve as precursors to language development. For instance, infants are intensely interested in human faces, and there is now evidence that the infant brain contains neurons that are specialized for the identification of human faces and for the recognition of affect in faces (Locke, 1993).

Language Areas in the Brain

Unlike our relatives the apes, humans have areas in the cerebral cortex that are known to be associated with language. The two hemispheres of the brain are not symmetrical (Geschwind, 1982). Most individuals, about 85 percent of the population, are right-handed, and almost all right-handers have their language functions represented in their left hemisphere. Of the left-handed population, perhaps half also have their language areas in the left hemisphere; therefore, the vast majority of the populace is **lateralized** for language in the left hemisphere. The right hemisphere, however, also participates in some aspects of language processing. For instance, recognition of the emotional tone of speech appears to be a right hemisphere function; moreover, when populations other than literate white males are studied, the cerebral asymmetry for language is less pronounced (Caplan, Lecours, & Smith, 1984).

New techniques, such as functional magnetic resonance imaging, have made it possible to study the normal brain in action. Shaywitz et al. (1995) reported finding sex differences in the neural organization of the brain for language. Females activate areas in both hemispheres during phonological processing, whereas males use a comparatively restricted area of the left hemisphere. Until recently, however, most of our information about specialized areas came from the study of what happens when the brain is injured, either through a traumatic accident or from a stroke, aneurysm, or other cardiovascular event. Damage to the language areas of the brain results in **aphasia,** a generalized communication disorder with varying characteristics depending on the site of the lesion (Gleason & Goodglass, 1984; Goodglass, 1981). There are at least three well-established major language areas in the left hemisphere (see Figure 1.1).

Broca's area in the left frontal region is very near to that part of the motor strip that controls the tongue and lips, and damage to Broca's area results in a typical aphasic syndrome, called Broca's aphasia, in which the patient has good comprehension but much difficulty with pronunciation and producing the little words of the language, such as articles and prepositions. Speech tends to be *telegraphic*—it contains only the most important words. For instance, when one patient seen in Boston was asked how he planned to spend the weekend at home, he replied, with labored articulation, "Boston College. Football. Saturday."

Wernicke's area is located in the posterior left temporal lobe, near the auditory association areas of the brain. Damage to Wernicke's area produces an aphasia that is characterized by fluent speech with many **neologisms** (nonsense words) and poor comprehension. One Wernicke's aphasic, when asked to name an ashtray, said, "That's a fremser." When he was later asked to point to the fremser, however, he had no idea what the examiner meant.

The **arcuate fasciculus** is a band of subcortical fibers that connects Wernicke's area with Broca's area. According to Geschwind's model (see Figure 1.1) if you ask someone to repeat what you say, the incoming message is processed in Wernicke's area and then sent out over the arcuate fasciculus to Broca's area, where it is programmed for production. Patients with lesions in the arcuate fasciculus are unable to repeat; their disorder is called **conduction aphasia.** There are also areas of the brain known to be associated with written language: Damage to the angular gyrus, for instance, impairs the ability to read.

A child of five or six who suffers left-brain damage will in all likelihood recover complete language. However, adults who become aphasic are liable to remain so if they do not recover in the first half-year after their injury.

Specialized language areas of the brain are found in adults, but there is evidence that in young children either the areas are not yet so firmly specialized or the nonlanguage hemisphere can take over in case of damage to the dominant hemisphere. The brains of infants are not fully formed and organized at birth. The brains of newborns have many fewer synapses (connections) than those of adults. By the age of about two, the number of synapses reaches adult levels, and then increases rapidly between the ages of four and ten, far exceeding adult levels. During this period of synaptic growth, there is a concurrent pruning process as connections that do not get used die off. This

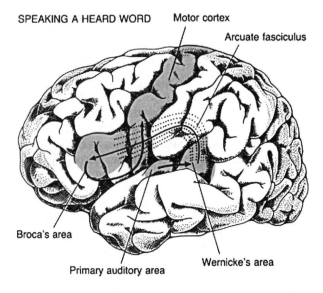

SPEAKING A HEARD WORD
Motor cortex
Arcuate fasciculus
Broca's area
Primary auditory area
Wernicke's area

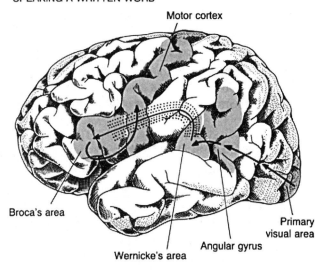

SPEAKING A WRITTEN WORD
Motor cortex
Broca's area
Primary visual area
Angular gyrus
Wernicke's area

Figure 1.1

Language areas in the brain. When a word is heard (upper diagram), the sensation from the ears is received by the primary auditory cortex, but the word cannot be understood until the signal has been processed in Wernicke's area nearby. If the word is to be spoken, some representation of it is thought to be transmitted from Wernicke's area to Broca's area, through a bundle of nerve fibers called the arcuate fasciculus. In Broca's area the word evokes a detailed program for articulation, which is supplied to the face area of the motor cortex. The motor cortex in turn drives the muscles of the lips, the tongue, the larynx, and so on. When a written word is read (lower diagram), the sensation is first registered by the primary visual cortex. It is then thought to be relayed to the angular gyrus, which associates the visual form of the word with the corresponding auditory pattern in Wernicke's area. Speaking the word then draws on the same systems of neurons as before. (Adapted from "Specializations of the Human Brain," by Norman Geschwind. Copyright © 1979 by Scientific American, Inc. All rights reserved.)

process may help to explain the neurological bases of sensitive or critical periods in development. If, for instance, an infant does not hear language or does not establish an emotional bond with an adult, the neural connections that underlie language and emotion may be weakened. By the age of fifteen or sixteen the number of synapses has returned to adult levels.

Special Characteristics

In examining the attempts to teach language to apes, we saw that language is probably species unique; the specialized areas of the brain contribute to that uniqueness. Human beings, of course, also have unique cognitive abilities and unique social settings in which to acquire language. These are discussed in subsequent chapters—the intent here is to describe briefly the neuroanatomical foundations that make language acquisition possible. As Eric Lenneberg (1967) pointed out, language development in humans is associated with other maturational events. The appearance of language is a developmental milestone, roughly correlated with the onset of walking. In addition to possessing specialized brain structures, humans, unlike other creatures, have a long list of specializations in such things as the development of their vocal cords and larynxes and the ability to coordinate phonation with breathing and swallowing. Humans perform a remarkably complex set of actions when they engage in everyday activities, such as having a talk over lunch. Lenneberg (1967) cited a number of additional features as evidence that language is specific to our species and uniform across the species in its major characteristics.

1. *The onset of speech is regular.* The order of appearance of developmental milestones, including speech, is regular in the species—it is not affected by culture or the language to be learned.

2. *Speech is not suppressible.* Normal children learn to talk if they are in contact with older speakers. The wide variations that exist within and across cultures have all provided suitable environments for children to learn language.

3. *Language cannot be taught to other species.* Lenneberg made this claim in the 1960s, before there were results from the chimpanzee (and parrot) studies, and time may have proven him right. However, it is also clear that chimpanzees can be taught sign language comparable to the language of young children; and thus this claim depends on only one definition of language.

4. *Languages everywhere have certain universals.* They are structured in accordance with principles of human cognition, and any human can learn any language. At the same time, there are universal constraints on the kinds of rules that children can learn. The universals that are found in all languages include phonology, grammar, and semantics. These systematic aspects of language, along with another universal, the existence of pragmat-

ics (social rules for language use), provide the research arena for developmental psycholinguistics.

The Structure of Language: Learning the System

Competence and Performance

A speaker who knows the syntactic rules of a language is said to have *linguistic competence*. Competence in this case refers to the inner knowledge of the rules, not to the way the person speaks on any particular occasion. The expression of the rules in everyday speech is *performance*. In the normal course of events, speakers produce errors, false starts, slips of the tongue, and utterances flawed in various other ways. These are performance errors and are not thought to reflect the speakers' underlying competence. There is also a general assumption among linguists that within a given linguistic community, all adults who are native speakers of the language, and not neurologically impaired in some way, share linguistic competence; this claim, however, has never been substantiated. It is possible to find out a great deal about adults' syntax by asking them to judge the grammatical acceptability of a sentence. However, in studying children, researchers must either rely on performance for clues to competence or design clever experiments to probe inner knowledge, since young children are not able to discuss questions of "grammaticality."

When children learn language, what is it that they must learn? Language has many subsystems having to do with sound, grammar, meaning, vocabulary, and knowing the right way to say something on a particular occasion in order to accomplish a specific purpose. Knowing the language entails knowing its **phonology, morphology, syntax,** and **semantics,** as well as its *pragmatics*. The speaker who knows all this has acquired *communicative competence* (Hymes, 1972).

Phonology

What are the sounds of English? Although we all speak the language, without specific training it would be difficult to list all of the sounds we make when we speak, and even more difficult to list the rules for their combination. Phonology includes all of the important sounds, the rules for combining them to make words, and such things as the stress and intonation patterns that accompany them. If you have studied foreign languages, you know that there are many different sounds used in the languages of the world and that any given language uses only a subset of the possibilities. Each language has its own set of important sounds, which are actually categories of sounds that include a number of variations. For instance, in English we pronounce the sound

/t/ many different ways: at the beginning of a word like *top* it is pronounced with a strong aspiration, or puff of air (you can check this by holding the back of your hand near your mouth and vigorously saying *top*). We pronounce a word like *stop* without the puff of air, unaspirated. Some speakers produce a different, unreleased /t/ when they say a word like *hat* at the end of a sentence: They leave their tongues in place at the point of articulation. Many speakers pronounce an even different kind of /t/ in a word like *Manhattan* by releasing the air through their noses at the end. A phonetician would hear these /t/ sounds as four different sounds: aspirated, unaspirated, unreleased, and nasally released. But for untrained English speakers, these are all just one sound. A group of similar sounds that are regarded as all the same by the speakers of a language are called phonemes. The different /t/ sounds just described are all part of one /t/ phoneme in English. In Hindi and many other Indian languages, the aspirated and unaspirated versions of /t/ are heard and treated as very different sounds, two different phonemes.

Children have to learn to recognize and produce the phonemes of their own language and to combine those phonemes into words and sentences with the right sorts of intonational patterns. Some parts of the system, such as consonant-vowel combinations, are acquired early on. Others are not acquired until well into the elementary school years: for instance, the ability to distinguish between the stress patterns of *hot dog* (frankfurter, with mustard) and *hot dog* (Weimaraner, with leash) when the words are presented without a context (Atkinson-King, 1973). The phonological tasks that face a young child can vary considerably from language to language. English and other Germanic languages, for instance, have quite complicated rules for the combination of consonants: We have many words like *risks* or *lengthy* that pose a challenge to anyone learning English. By contrast, Japanese has very few consonant clusters.

English has some sounds rarely found in other languages of the world, such as the *th* sound in *this;* but Czech has an even rarer sound, the medial sound /ř/ in the name *Dvořak,* which is a combination of an /r/ trilled on the tip of the tongue and the /ž/ sound in *azure,* said at the same time. Many African languages contain phonemic clicks rather similar to the sounds we make in English when we say what is written as "tsk tsk" or when we encourage a horse to go faster. In some languages tone is a phoneme: In Chinese, a rising or falling tone on a word can change its meaning entirely. When the tones are produced correctly, the sentence "Mama ma ma ma?" means "Did mother chide the horse?"

Morphology

When a new word, such as *glitch* or *dweeb,* comes into the English language, adult speakers can immediately tell what its plural is; they do not have to look it up in a dictionary or consult with an expert. They are able to pluralize a word that they have never heard before because they know the English inflectional morphological system. A **morpheme** is the smallest unit of meaning in a language; it cannot be broken into any smaller parts that have meaning. Words can consist of one or more morphemes. The words *cat* and *danger* each consist of one morpheme, which is called a **free morpheme** because it can stand alone. **Bound morphemes,** on the other hand, cannot stand alone and are always found attached to free morphemes; they appear affixed to free morphemes as prefixes, suffixes, or within the word as infixes. *Happiness, unclear,* and *singing* contain the bound morphemes *-ness, -un,* and *-ing.* Bound morphemes can be used to change one word into another word that may be a different part of speech; for instance, *-ness* turns the adjective *happy* into the noun *happiness.* In this case, they are called **derivational morphemes** because they can be used to derive new words.

Other bound morphemes do not change the basic word's meaning so much as they modify it to indicate such things as tense, person, number, case, and gender. These variations on a basic word are inflections, and the morphemes that accomplish these changes are inflectional morphemes. Languages like Latin, Russian, and Hungarian are highly inflected. The verb *to love (amare)* in Latin has six separate forms in the present tense.

amo I love	*amamus* we love
amas you love (sing.)	*amatis* you love (pl.)
amat he loves	*amant* they love

Compared with Latin, English has few verb inflections in the present tense: an added *-s* for the third person (he *loves*) and no inflection for other persons (I, we, you, they *love*). Latin indicates the subject and object of its sentences using case inflections—*agricola amat puellam* and *puellam amat agricola* both mean "the farmer loves the girl." The endings of the words mark the subject and the object. English does not have case endings on its nouns: Whether the girl loves the farmer or the farmer loves the girl is indicated entirely by word order. Grammar teachers, perhaps influenced by their knowledge of Latin, have tended to confuse the issue in English by referring to nouns as being in the subjective or objective case when, in fact, there are no separate noun case forms in English. Pronouns, on the other hand, have subjective, objective, and possessive forms: *I, me,* and *my.* Even with pronouns, however, word order is more important in English than it is in Latin—on hearing the sentence "Me saw it," most English speakers assume that "me" did the seeing, however ungrammatical the phrase.

English inflectional morphology includes the progressive of the verb (e.g., *singing*); the past, pronounced with /d/, /t/ or /əd/, *(played, hopped, landed);* and the third person singular verb and the noun plural and possessive, all of which use /z/, /s/, or /əz/ in spoken language *(dogs, cats, watches).* Whether one says, "He dogs my steps" (verb), "It's the dog's dish" (possessive), or, "I have ten dogs" (plural), the inflected form is pronounced in exactly the same way. The forms of the inflections vary depending on the last sound of the word being inflected, and, as stated earlier, there is a complex set of rules that adult speakers know (at some level) that enables them to make a plural or past tense of a word that they have never heard before.

One task for the student of language development is to determine whether children have knowledge of morphology and, if so, how it is acquired and to what extent it resembles the rule system that adults follow.

Syntax

The syntactic system contains the rules for how to combine words into phrases and sentences and how to transform sentences into other sentences. A competent speaker can take a basic sentence like "The cat bites the dog" and make a number of transformations of it: "The cat bit the dog," "The cat didn't bite the dog," "Did the cat bite the dog?" and "Wasn't the dog bitten by the cat?" Knowledge of the syntactic system allows the speaker to generate an almost endless number of new sentences and to recognize those that are not grammatically acceptable. If you heard a nonsense sentence like "The gorpy wug wasn't miggled by the mimsy zibber," you could not know what happened because the vocabulary is strange. On the other hand, the morphology and syntax of the sentence convey a great deal of information, and with this information you could make a number of new, perfectly grammatical sentences: "The wug is gorpy," "The zibber did not miggle the wug," and "The zibber is mimsy."

There is a great deal of controversy among researchers as to whether young children just learning language are acquiring syntactic structures, that is, grammatical rules, or whether it is more reasonable to characterize their early utterances in terms of the semantic relations they are trying to express. The child who says, "Doggie eat lunch," can be said to have learned to produce subject-verb-object constructions and to be following English syntactic rules specifying that the subject comes first in active sentences. (Even very young children do not say, "Lunch eat doggie.") To describe the language of young children, however, it is probably more useful to note the kinds of semantic relations the children are using. In this case the child is expressing her knowledge that an action is taking place and that there is an agent and an object.

Once children begin to produce longer sentences, however, they add the grammatical words of the language and begin to build sentences according to syntactic rules. They learn how to make *negatives, questions, compound sentences, passives,* and *imperatives.* Later, they add very complex structures, including embedded forms. The child who early on was limited to sentences like "Doggie eat lunch" can eventually comprehend and produce "The lunch that Grandpa cooked the cleaning lady was eaten by the dog" in full confidence that the household helper was neither cooked by Grandpa nor eaten by Bluto.

Semantics

Semantic acquisition refers to the acquisition of vocabulary and the meanings associated with words. Word meanings are complicated to learn; words are related to one another in complex networks, and awareness of words comes later than does word use. A very young child may use a word that occurs in adult language, but that word does not mean exactly the same thing, nor does it have the same internal status for the child as it does for the adult (Clark, 1993). Two-year-olds who say "doggie," for instance, may call sheep, cows, cats, and horses "doggie," or they may use the word in reference to a particular dog, without knowing that it refers to a whole class of animals. Vocabulary is structured hierarchically, and words are attached to one another in semantic networks. Dogs are a class of animals, and the adult who knows the meaning of *dog* also knows, for instance, that it belongs to a group known as domestic animals, it is a pet, it is related to wolves, it is animate, etc. Studying semantic development in children involves examining the ways in which they acquire the semantic system, beginning with simple vocabulary. Ultimately, it includes studying their metalinguistic knowledge, which enables them to notice the words in their language and comment on them. A young child does not know what a word is, but by the time children are in the primary grades, they not only notice words, they can provide definitions and tell such things as what their favorite words are.

Pragmatics

Linguistic competence resides in knowing how to construct grammatically acceptable sentences. Language, however, must be used in a social setting, to accomplish various ends. Speakers who know how to use language *appropriately* have more than linguistic competence; they have communicative competence, a term first used by Dell Hymes (1972). *Pragmatics* refers to the use of language to express one's intentions and get things done in the world. Even children at the one-word stage use language to accomplish various pragmatic ends; John Dore (1978), for instance, found that such children used their single words to ask, demand, and label. Adult pragmatics may include such additional functions as denying, refusing, blaming, offering condolences, flattering, and a host of others.

Communicative competence includes being able to express one's pragmatic intent appropriately in varying social situations. The importance of knowing the right forms becomes obvious when social rules are violated. Consider the use of directives. If you are seated in the aisle seat of a train, next to a stranger, and you are cold because the window is open, you can express your pragmatic intent in a syntactically correct sentence: "Shut that window." This could lead to a hostile reaction or, at the very least, to the impression that you are a rude person. If, instead, you said, "I wonder if you would mind shutting the window?" compliance and the beginning of a pleasant conversation would probably follow. Knowing the politeness rules of language is part of communicative competence.

Research on pragmatics examines the way that children learn to use language appropriately in various social situations. Pragmatics includes important topics, such as the ability to make conversation. Pellegrini, Brody, and Stoneman (1987) studied the ways that children learn to make appropriate conversations with their parents. These researchers used a model provided by the philosopher Herbert Grice.

Grice (1975) provided a framework for the study of conversations by setting forth a number of cooperative principles or maxims that successful conversationalists must obey. These *conversational principles* include:

1. *Quantity.* Be as informative as necessary, but not overly so. For instance, if someone asks a child what she would like to drink with dinner, she must know that it suffices to say, "Orange juice, please," and that it would be inappropriate to say, "Approximately eight ounces of juice squeezed from several oranges and placed in a glass here on the table at the right of my plate." Young children are, of course, likely to give too little rather than too much information.

2. *Quality.* This maxim requires that what one says be the truth. Children must learn that their interlocutors expect them not to lie.

3. *Relevance.* Contributions to the conversation are expected to be relevant. If a child responds to the question "What do you like for lunch?" by saying, "I like my kitty," she is violating the relevance principle (or exhibiting serious antisocial tendencies).

4. *Manner.* Speakers are expected to take their turns in a timely fashion and to present their propositions in a logical order. It is a violation of this principle, for instance, to say, "We put on our pajamas and took a bath," since presumably bathing precedes putting on pajamas.

Adults, of course, violate these principles in order to achieve certain very human ends: to be ironic, for instance, or to make a joke, or perhaps to be deceptive or insulting. Every type of interaction between individuals requires observance of pragmatic conventions, and adults do not leave children's development of these rules to chance—whereas they may not correct syntactic violations except in the most superficial cases (see Chapter 5), they are active participants in their children's pragmatic socialization (Becker, 1994).

Just as there are phonological and grammatical rules, there are also rules for the use of language in social context. They are governed by such variables as the topic, the channel of communication (e.g., face-to-face, on the telephone, or over a CB radio), and the social situation—one might speak quite differently about the same topic at a funeral than at a wedding. There are also a number of speaker/hearer characteristics that affect the form of the communication; these include gender, age, rank, social class, and degree of familiarity. Mature language users have all of these variables under control. They know how to speak like men or women, to conduct discourse, to speak in appropriate ways to different people. They can talk baby talk to babies and be formal and deferential when appearing in court. All of these are part of communicative competence, which is the goal of language development.

The Study of Language Development

Historical Trends in Child Language Study

Probably the first recorded account of a language acquisition study is found in the work of the Greek historian Herodotus, who was a contemporary of the playwright Sophocles. Herodotus, sometimes called the father of history, lived from about 484 to 425 B.C. In Book 11 of his *History*, he relates the story of the ancient Egyptian king Psammetichus, who wanted to prove that the Egyptians were the original human race.

In order to do this, Psammetichus ordered a shepherd to raise two children, caring for their needs but not speaking to them. "His object herein was to know, after the indistinct babblings of infancy were over, what word they would first articulate." Presumably, Psammetichus believed that the children would develop the language of the oldest group of humans all by themselves. This is perhaps the strongest version of an innatist theory of language development that one could have: Babies arrive in the world with a specific language wired into their brains.

When the two children were about two years old, the shepherd went to their quarters one day. They ran up to him, with their hands outstretched, saying "Becos." Unfortunately for the Egyptians, *becos* was not a word that anyone recognized. The king, according to Herodotus, asked around the kingdom and eventually was told that *becos* meant "bread" in the Phrygian language, whereupon the Egyptians gave up their claim to being the oldest race of humans and decided that they were in *second* place, behind the Phrygians.

Even though interest in language development has ancient roots, the systematic study of children's language is new to our times, in part because the science of linguistics, with its special analytic techniques, has come of age in our own century. In earlier times, the structural nature of language was not well understood, and what studies there were tended to concentrate on the kinds of things that children said rather than on their acquisition of productive linguistic subsystems.

Studies in the Late Nineteenth and Early Twentieth Century

There were many studies of children, including notes on their language, published in Germany, France, and England during the latter half of the nineteenth century and the early years of the twentieth century. One of the main early figures in the United States in the field of developmental psychology, G. Stanley Hall, taught at Clark University in Worcester, Massachusetts. Hall (1907) was interested in "the content of children's minds," and he had been led to study children's language by the German philosopher Wilhelm Wundt. Hall, in turn, inspired a school of American students of child language (Bar-Adon & Leopold, 1971).

The kinds of questions that child language researchers asked during this period were primarily related to philosophical inquiries into human nature. (This was true of Charles Darwin, 1877, who kept careful diaries on the language development of one of his sons.) Many of these early investigations included valuable insights into language. (A number of such studies are summarized in Bar-Adon and Leopold, 1971.) The early studies were almost invariably in the form of diaries, and were typically observations of the authors' own children. Notable exceptions were studies of feral or isolated children who had failed to acquire language. Just as in antiquity, there was philosophical interest in the effects of isolation on language development; that interest has been sustained to the present day: *The Wild Boy of Aveyron,* a landmark study of a feral child, Victor, was written in the eighteenth century (Lane, 1979), and the study of Genie, an American girl who was kept isolated from other humans, was published not long ago (Curtiss, 1977; Rymer, 1993).

During the first half of the twentieth century, many psychologists still kept diary records of their children. In the educational world, children's language was studied in order to arrive at norms, delineate gender and social class differences, and pinpoint the causes and cures of developmental difficulties. Educational psychologists frequently used group tests with large numbers of children, and there was a great interest in such things as the average sentence length used by children at different grade levels, or the kinds of errors they made in grammar or pronunciation (McCarthy, 1954).

Contemporary Research

The mid-1950s saw a revolution in child language studies. Work on descriptive linguistics (Gleason, 1955) and the early work of Noam Chomsky (1957) provided new models of language for researchers to explore. At the same time, a behaviorist theory of language put forth by B. F. Skinner (1957) inspired other groups of investigators to design studies aimed at testing this learning theory.

Psycholinguistics came into being as a field when linguists and psychologists combined the techniques of their disciplines to investigate whether the systems described by the linguist had psychological reality in the minds of speakers. The linguistic description of English might, for instance, point out that the plural of words ending in /s/ or /z/ is formed by adding /əz/, for example, *kiss* and *kisses*. A task for the psycholinguist was to demonstrate that the linguistic description matched what speakers actually do, that speakers have a "rule" for the formation of the plural that is isomorphic (i.e., identical in form) with the linguist's descriptive rule. If speakers merely memorized the plural of each new word in their lexicon or vocabulary, there would be no evidence of internal rules.

In the decade of the 1960s, after the powerful, transformational model of Chomsky became widely known, there was an explosion of research into children's acquisition of syntax. The 1960s were characterized by studies of grammar; many projects studied a small number of children over a period of time, writing grammars of the children's developing language. At Harvard University, for instance, a group of researchers, many of whom were to become prominent individually, worked with Roger Brown (1973) on a project that studied the language of three children called Adam, Eve, and Sarah. These children were visited once a month in their homes by researchers who made tape recordings of their speech. The recordings were brought back to the laboratory and transcribed, and the resulting transcriptions were studied by a team of faculty and graduate students that met in a weekly seminar (DeCuevas, 1990).

As the 1960s drew to a close, the primacy of syntax in research gave way to a broadening interest that included the context in which children's language emerges and an emphasis on the kinds of semantic relations children are trying to express in their early utterances. The early 1970s saw a spate of studies on the language addressed to children; many of these were conducted to shed light on the innateness controversy. Researchers wanted to know whether children had to discover the rules of language all by themselves, or whether adults provided them with help or even with language learning lessons.

Studies of the 1980s and thus far in the 1990s include all of the traditional topics: phonology, morphology, syntax, semantics, and pragmatics. There is also growing interest in cross-cultural research in language development, and in understanding how language development interfaces with other aspects of children's social and psychological development; in acquiring a language, children become members of a society, with all of its unique cultural practices and belief systems. Cross-cultural work has shown, for instance, that in a nonliterate society such as that of Gypsies in Hungary, parents' speech to children has special features that serve to preserve traditions and inculcate cultural values—for example, parents tell even infants detailed stories about what their future life will be like (Réger & Gleason, 1991).

Social class and gender differences in language, stylistic variation in acquisition and use, the use of language in poetry and metaphor and in jokes and games, and the language addressed to children are examples of topics found in current journals devoted to the various branches of linguistics. Many of these topics are also explored in later chapters of this book.

Research Methods

Equipment

Modern technology has made it possible to collect accurate data on children's everyday use of language. When developmental psycholinguistics was born in the 1950s, technology was very limited, and researchers had to rely on large reel-to-reel tape recorders and handwritten notes when they collected their data. There were no photocopy machines. Cassette audio recorders and palm-held video recorders have greatly simplified data collection, and computers have made analysis easier.

Studies of phonology require especially sensitive recording equipment, and must frequently use sophisticated laboratory hardware, which is now often computerized as well. Other studies, however, can usually be conducted with easily acquired equipment. A good cassette recorder is sufficient for most work, and if there is a great deal of data, a cassette transcriber is an invaluable aid. Some studies require a visual record; if, for instance, the researcher is interested in the gestural accompaniments of early language or the gaze behavior of subjects, low-light video cameras and lightweight video recording equipment are now widely available. This equipment makes it possible to film in subjects' homes with a minimum of intrusion. Video makes it possible to study the context of language acquisition. Most researchers use a back-up tape recorder in addition to their video equipment. Because the presence of equipment and observers will invariably have some effect on the behavior of subjects, it is possible in some naturalistic studies to leave a recorder with the subjects, instructing the subjects (or their parents) to turn it on at specified times.

Regardless of the method of recording, it is necessary to make a transcription of the data for analysis. This involves writing out as exactly as possible everything that is said on the tape. Transcripts can then be prepared in such a way that computer analyses are possible (see Figure 1.2).

One of the most significant developments in child language research is the creation of a computerized child language data base available to researchers. The Child Language Data Exchange System (CHILDES) was put into operation in 1984 at Carnegie Mellon University under the direction of Brian MacWhinney and Catherine Snow. Many powerful computer programs (CLAN, or Child Language Analysis programs) are available, along with data, from CHILDES (MacWhinney, 1991). They include programs that operate on any or all speakers' output and can automatically derive the mean length of utterance (see Chapter 5), a total list of words used, as well as their frequency, and other data of immense value to the language researcher.

Data from many studies are available; there are separate directories containing transcripts of speech from English-speaking, non-English-speaking, and atypically developing children. Older studies, such as Brown's famous work on Adam, Eve, and Sarah from the 1960s, have been optically scanned and entered, thus making these data available to anyone who wants them. This system continues to collect data from researchers all over the world. Its advantages are that it allows (1) data sharing among researchers, who can test their hypotheses on many more subjects; (2) increased precision and standardization in coding; and (3) automation of many coding procedures.

Methods

Language development studies can be either *cross-sectional* or *longitudinal* in their design. Cross-sectional studies use two or more groups of subjects. If, for instance, you wanted to study the development of the negative between the ages of two and

```
@Begin
@Participants:  CHI Andy Child, MOT Mother, FAT Father
@Date:          7-JUL-1995
@Filename:      ANDY.CHA
@Situation:     Home Dinner Conversation
*CHI:           I-'m hungry
*FAT:           you are?
*CHI:           I-'m gonna eat my spaghetti.
*CHI:           get big and strong.
*MOT:           so you-'ll be tall-er?
*FAT:           how big and strong do you want to be?
*CHI:           I-'m get-ing big-er and big-er and big-er.
*FAT:           and big-er and big-er.
*FAT:           how big are you go-ing to be?
*FAT:           uh oh.
*FAT:           do you want any sauce?
*FAT:           hm?
*CHI:           not this time.
*FAT:           you do-'nt want it this time?
*CHI:           I want some cheese.
*MOT:           is that gonna be enough for you?
*CHI:           I think so.
*MOT:           you can have more.
*CHI:           okay.
@End
```

Figure 1.2

Sample transcript in CHAT format. *This transcript can be analyzed by a variety of CLAN computer programs that can automatically compute MLU, list all vocabulary by speaker, and derive many standardized measures.*

four, you could study a group of two-year-olds and a group of four-year-olds and then describe the differences in the two groups' use of negation.

Longitudinal studies follow individual subjects over time; one might study the same child's use of negatives at specified periods between the ages of two and four. Unless the researcher has ample funding, it is usually impossible to follow more than a few subjects in a longitudinal study.

Cross-sectional studies have the advantage of obtaining a great deal of data in a short time; one doesn't have to wait two years to get results. Having a sizable number of subjects also makes it more likely that the results of the study are generalizable to other children and not a reflection of the idiosyncratic behavior of a few. Longitudinal designs are used to study individuals over time when questions such as the persistence of traits or the effects of early experience are relevant. If, for instance, you wanted to know whether children who talk early also become early readers, you would have to use a longitudinal design. Longitudinal studies are expensive and time-consuming, and they depend on the willingness of subjects to be available for a period of weeks, months, or years. Their advantage is that they can provide fine and accurate data about what happens to individuals during the course of language development.

Both cross-sectional and longitudinal studies can be either *observational* or *experimental.* Observational studies involve a minimum of intrusion by the researcher. Naturalistic observational studies attempt to capture behavior as it occurs in real life; for instance, one might record and analyze family speech at the dinner table. Controlled observational studies can be carried out in various settings, including the laboratory; here the researcher provides certain constants for all subjects. Fathers might come to the laboratory with their daughters and be observed reading them a book provided by the researcher. Observational research can indicate what kinds of behaviors correlate with one another, but it cannot reveal which behavior might cause another.

Experimental studies involve some manipulation on the part of the researcher. In classic experimental designs, the researcher attempts to show that a particular manipulation causes a particular outcome. Typically, there is a *control group* of subjects that receives no special treatment, and an *experimental group* that receives the particular manipulation that the experimenter has chosen. If you wanted to see whether training makes a difference in the acquisition of the passive voice, for instance, you might take a group of thirty three-year-olds and randomly assign them to two groups, a control group and an experimental group of fifteen children each. The experimental group would receive training in the passive; the control group, no special treatment. Finally, both groups could be asked to describe some pictures they had never seen before, and differential use of the passive would be recorded. If the trained group used passives and the control group did not, there would be evidence that training causes accelerated acquisition of one aspect of grammar.

In addition to clear-cut observational and experimental methods, language development researchers use a variety of research techniques. These include *standard assessment measures,* in which subjects can be compared or evaluated on the basis of their responses to published standardized language tests. These are useful for indicating whether a subject is developing at a typical rate or whether some facet of development is out of line with the others.

Imitation is a technique used by many researchers—you simply ask the child to say what you say. Imitation reveals a great deal about children's language, since they typically cannot imitate sentences that are beyond their stage of development (Slobin,

1979). This is true of adults as well—try imitating a few sentences in Bulgarian the next time you meet someone from Sofia who is willing to say them to you.

Elicitation is a technique that works well when a particular language form is the target, and you want to give your subjects all the help they need (short of the answer itself). In investigating the plural through elicitation, you might show your subjects a picture, first of one and then of two birdlike creatures, and say, "This is a wug. Now there is another one. There are two of them. There are two...?" The subject obligingly fills in "wugs." This technique works well with aphasic patients, especially severe Broca's aphasics who have very little voluntary speech.

The *interview* is an old technique, but one that can be very effective if the researcher has the time to do more than ask a list of questions and fill in a form. Researchers of the Piagetian school frequently use an interview type called the *clinical method.* This is an open-ended interview in which the sequence of questions depends on the answers the subject has given. In studying metalinguistic awareness, the investigator might ask a series of questions, such as "Is *horse* a word? Why? (Or why not?) What is a word? How do you know? What is your favorite word? Why?" The choice of method depends very much on the theoretical inclination of the investigator. Every method that has been mentioned here, as well as a few that have not, appears in the pages that follow.

Summary

Babies seek the love and attention of their caregivers. Before they are even one year old, they are able to make fine discriminations among the speech sounds they hear, and they begin to communicate nonverbally with those around them. Young children acquire the basic components of their native language in just a few years: *phonology, morphology, semantics, syntax,* and *pragmatics.* By the time they are of school age they control all of the major grammatical and semantic features. Language development, however, proceeds throughout the life cycle; as individuals grow older, they acquire new skills at every stage of their lives, and in the declining years they are vulnerable to a specific set of language disabilities. To elucidate both the scope and the nature of language development, this book is written from a life-span perspective.

Babies begin to acquire language during their first months, long before they say their first words; language is built upon an affective prelinguistic communicative base. Midway through the first year, infants begin to babble, an event seen by many researchers as evidence of linguistic capacity. Near their first birthdays, infants say their first words. Early words, word meanings, and word combinations have universal characteristics, since toddlers' language is similar across cultures. Children's progress toward learning the particular grammatical structure of their own language follows a predictable order that is common to all children learning that language.

Although there are universal characteristics, there are also patterns of individual variation in language development. Different theories of language development emphasize *innate mechanisms; learning principles; cognitive prerequisites; information processing;* and *social interaction.*

During the school years, children perfect their knowledge of complex grammar, and they learn to use language in many different social situations. At the same time, they learn another major linguistic system: the written language. The demands of literacy remove a child's language from the here and now and emphasize *decontextualized language.* Not all children learn to read with ease.

Teenagers develop a distinct personal linguistic style, and young adults must acquire the linguistic register common to their occupations. With advancing age, numerous linguistic changes take place; there is some inevitable loss of word-finding ability, but vocabulary and narrative skill may improve.

Human language has special properties that have led many researchers to conclude that it is *species specific* and *species uniform.* Insects may have an elaborate communication system but their conversational topics are very limited, whereas humans can talk about any part of their experience. Sea mammals employ communicative systems of whistles and grunts, and many birds have been shown to have a variety of meaningful calls. None of these systems equals human language, however, which is *productive,* has *semanticity,* and offers the possibility of *displacement.*

During the past half-century, many researchers have turned their attention to primates in an attempt to discover whether language is really unique to humans or if it can be learned by other species. The early studies, which tried to teach spoken language to chimpanzees, showed conclusively that primates cannot speak as humans do. More recent studies have attempted to teach American Sign Language (ASL) to chimpanzees and have met with mixed results. The signing chimps appear to be responding at least in part to subtle cues from their trainers, but the question of the apes' potential is not completely settled. These studies have indicated that there are substantial similarities between very young children's and chimpanzees' abilities to engage in symbolic communication, and there is the possibility that the bonobo (pygmy chimpanzee) will reach new heights of linguistic achievement.

Language development requires social interaction, but spoken language in humans is possible only because we have evolved with specialized neural mechanisms that subserve language. These include special areas in the brain, such as *Broca's area, Wernicke's area,* and the *arcuate fasciculus.* Other evidence of humans' biological disposition for language includes the regular onset of speech and the facts that speech is not suppressible, language cannot be taught to other species, and languages everywhere have universals.

The study of language development includes research into major linguistic subsystems. The *phonological system* is composed of the significant sounds of the language and the rules for their combination, the *morphological system* includes the minimal units that carry meaning, *syntax* refers to the rules by which sentences are constructed in a given language, and the *semantic systems* contains the meanings of words and the relationships between them. Finally, to function in society, speakers must know the *pragmatic rules* for language use. Individuals must be able to comprehend and produce all of these systems in order to attain *communicative competence.*

Although interest in language development has ancient roots, the scientific study of this subject began in the 1950s, with the appearance of new linguistic and psychological theories of language that gave birth to the combined discipline now known as *developmental psycholinguistics.* Developmental psycholinguists use all of the research techniques, designs, and resources employed by psychologists and linguists, as well as a few that are unique, such as a new computerized data bank of child language materials.

Key Words

American Sign Language (ASL)	metalinguist awareness
aphasia	morpheme
arcuate fasciculus	morphology
autism	neologisms
bound morpheme	overlaid function
Broca's area	overregularized
child-directed speech (CDS)	phonology
communicative competence	pragmatics
comprehension	production
conduction aphasia	semantic development
decontextualized language	semantics
derivational morpheme	species specific
dyslexia	species uniform
free morpheme	specific language impairment
innate	speech acts
internalized representation	syntax
lateralized	telegraphic
linguistic competence	Wernicke's area

Suggested Projects

1. Choose three related articles on language development from the *Journal of Child Language,* or from another journal such as *Child Development.* Write an introduction, explaining what the major questions of the research are, and then, for each article, describe the methods used by the authors, the subject population, any special equipment that was needed, and the nature of the results. In a separate discussion section, compare the results of the studies, and suggest other ways that the same question could be explored.

2. Tape-record a half-hour sample of a mother or father interacting with a one- or two-year-old child who does not yet combine words. At the end of the session, have a brief discussion with the parent about the child for about five minutes. Transcribe the entire tape. Analyze and compare the parent's speech to the child and speech to you in terms of (a) the average length of sentence, (b) repetitions, (c) the vocabulary used by the parent. Describe and categorize the vocabulary used by the child.

3. Read papers by the Premacks, Rumbaughs, and Terrace on their studies of the symbolic capacities of chimpanzees. Summarize the claims that are made for these apes, and provide a critique.

Suggested Readings

Brown, R. W. (1970). The first sentences of child and chimpanzee. In R. W. Brown (Ed.), *Psycholinguistics.* New York: Macmillan.

Curtiss, S. (1977). *Genie: A psycholinguistic study of a modern day "wild" child.* New York: Academic Press.

Diamond, J. (1992). *The third chimpanzee: The evolution and future of the human animal.* New York: Basic Books.

Gardner, R. A., & Gardner, B. T. (1980). Two comparative psychologists look at language acquisition. In K. E. Nelson (Ed.), *Children's language* (Vol. 2). New York: Gardner Press.

Geschwind, N. (1982). Specializations of the human brain. In W. S.-Y. Wang (Ed.), *Human communication: Language and its psychobiological bases.* San Francisco: W. H. Freeman.

Greenfield, P. M., & Savage-Rumbaugh, E. S. (1991). Imitation, grammatical development, and the invention of protogrammar by an ape. In N. Krasnegor, D. M. Rumbaugh, M. Studdert-Kennedy, & R. L. Schiefelbusch (Eds.), *Biological and behavioral determinants of language development.* Hillsdale, NJ: Lawrence Erlbaum.

Lane, H. (1979). *The wild boy of Aveyron.* Cambridge, MA: Harvard University Press.

Terrace, H. S. (1980). *Nim: A chimpanzee who learned sign language.* New York: Knopf.

References

Atkinson-King, K. (1973). Children's acquisition of phonological stress contrasts. UCLA Working Papers in Phonetics (Department of Linguistics), 25.

Bar-Adon, A., & Leopold, W. (1971). *Child language: A book of readings.* Englewood Cliffs, NJ: Prentice-Hall.

Becker, J. A. (1994). Pragmatic socialization: Parental input to preschoolers. *Discourse Processes, 17,* 131–148.

Berko, J. (1958). The child's learning of English morphology. *Word, 14,* 150–177.

Blake, J., & Boysson-Bardies, B. de (1992). Patterns in babbling: a cross linguistic study. *Journal of Child Language, 19,* 51–75.

Bloom, L. (1970). *Language development. Form and function in emerging grammars.* Cambridge, MA: MIT Press.

Bonvillian, J. D., & Patterson, F. G. (1993). Early sign language acquisition in children and gorillas: Vocabulary content and sign iconicity. *First Language, 13,* 315–338.

Boysson-Bardies, B. de, & Vihman, M. M. (1991). Adaptation to language: Evidence from babbling and first words in four languages. *Language, 67,* 297–319.

Brown, R. W. (1970). The first sentences of child and chimpanzee. In R. Brown (Ed.), *Psycholinguistics.* New York: Macmillan.

Brown, R. W. (1973). *A first language.* Cambridge, MA: Harvard University Press.

Caplan, D., Lecours, A., & Smith, A. (Eds.). (1984). *Biological perspectives on language.* Cambridge, MA: MIT Press.

Clark, E. V. (1973). What's in a word? On the child's acquisition of semantics in his first language. In T. E. Moore (Ed.), *Cognitive Development and the Acquisition of Language.* New York: Academic Press.

Clark, E. V. (1993). *The lexicon in acquisition.* Cambridge, UK: Cambridge University Press.

Chomsky, N. (1957). *Syntactic structures.* The Hague: Mouton.

Chomsky, N. (1965). *Aspects of the theory of syntax.* Cambridge, MA: MIT Press.

Curtiss, S. (1977). *Genie: A psycholinguistic study of a modern day "wild" child.* New York: Academic Press.

Darwin, C. (1877). A biographical sketch of an infant. *Mind, 2,* 285–294.

DeCuevas, J. (1990, September-October). "No, she holded them loosely." *Harvard Magazine,* 61–67.

Diamond, J. 1992. *The third chimpanzee: The evolution and future of the human animal.* New York: Basic Books.

Dore, J. (1978). Variation in preschool children's conversational performances. In K. Nelson (Ed.), *Children's language* (Vol. 1). New York: Gardner Press.

Dromi, E., & Berman, R. (1982). A morphemic measure of early language development: Data from modern Hebrew. *Journal of Child Language, 2,* 403–424.

Eimas, P. D. (1975). Auditory and phonetic coding of the cues for speech: Discrimination of the /r-l/ distinction by young infants. *Perception and Psychophysics, 18,* 341–347.

Erikson, E. (1959). Identity and the life cycle. *Psychological Issues, 1,* 1–171.

Fischer, S. (1993). The study of sign languages and linguistic theory. In C. Otero (Ed.), *Noam Chomsky: Critical assessments.* London: Routledge.

Gardner, R. A., & Gardner, B. T. (1969). Teaching sign language to a chimpanzee. *Science, 165,* 664–672.

Gardner, R. A., & Gardner, B. T. (1980). Two comparative psychologists look at language acquisition. In K. E. Nelson (Ed.), *Children's language* (Vol. 2). New York: Gardner Press.

Gardner, R. A., & Gardner, B. T. (1984a). A vocabulary test for chimpanzees. *Journal of Comparative Psychology,* 381–404.

Gardner, R. A., & Gardner, B. T. (1984b). Signs of intelligence in cross fostered chimpanzees, *Philosophical Transactions in the Royal Society of London, B,* 1–34.

Geschwind, N. (1982). Specializations of the brain. In W. S.-Y. Wang (Ed.), *Human communication: Language and its psychobiological bases.* San Francisco: W. H. Freeman.

Gleason, H. A. (1955). *An introduction to descriptive linguistics.* New York: Henry Holt.

Gleason, J. Berko, & Goodglass, H. (1984). Some neurological and linguistic accompaniments of the fluent and nonfluent aphasias. *Topics in Language Disorders, 4,* 71–81.

Goodglass, H. (1981). The syndromes of aphasia: Similarities and differences in neurolinguistic features. *Topics in Language Disorders, 1,* 1–14.

Greenfield, P. M., & Savage-Rumbaugh, E. S. (1991). Imitation, grammatical development, and the invention of protogrammar by an ape. In N. Krasnegor, D. M. Rumbaugh, M. Studdert-Kennedy, & R. L. Schiefelbusch (Eds.), *Biological and behavioral determinants of language development.* Hillsdale, NJ: Lawrence Erlbaum.

Grice, H. P. (1975). Logic and conversation. In P. Cole & J. Morgan (Eds.), *Syntax and semantics* (Vol. 3). New York: Academic Press.

Hall, G. S. (1907). *Aspects of child life and education.* New York: Appleton.

Hayes, C. (1951). *The ape in our house.* New York: Harper.

Herman, L. (1981). Cognitive characteristics of dolphins. In L. Herman (Ed.), *Cetacean behavior.* New York: Wiley.

Hymes, D. (1972). On communicative competence. In J. Pride & J. Holmes (Eds.), *Sociolinguistics.* Hammondsworth, G. B.: Penguin.

Jakobson, R. (1968). *Child language, aphasia, and phonological universals.* The Hague: Mouton.

Kellogg, W. N. (1980). Communication and language in the home raised chimpanzee. In T. Sebeok & J. Umiker Sebeok (Eds.), *Speaking of apes.* New York: Plenum Press.

Klima, E. S., & Bellugi, U. (1972). The signs of language in child and chimpanzee. In R. Alloway, L. Krames, & P. Pliner (Eds.), *Communication and affect. A comparative approach.* New York: Academic Press.

Klima, E. S., & Bellugi, U. (1979). *The signs of language.* Cambridge, MA: Harvard University Press.

Kuhl, P. K., Williams, K. A., Lacerda, F., Stevens, K. N., & Lindblom, B. (1992). Linguistic experience alters phonetic perception in infants by 6 months of age. *Science, 255,* 606—608.

Lane, H. (1979). *The wild boy of Aveyron.* Cambridge, MA: Harvard University Press.

Lenneberg, E. (1967). *The biological foundations of language.* New York: Wiley.

Lieven, E. (1978). Conversations between mothers and young children: Individual differences and their possible implications for the study of language learning. In N. Waterson & C. E. Snow (Eds.), *The development of communication.* New York: Wiley.

Locke, J. L. (1990). Structure and stimulation in the ontogeny of spoken language. *Developmental Psychobiology, 23(7),* 621–644.

Locke, J. L. (1993). *The child's path to spoken language.* Cambridge, MA: Harvard University Press.

Lorenz, K. (1971). *Studies in animal behavior.* Cambridge, MA: Harvard University Press.

MacWhinney, B. (1991). *The CHILDES Project. Computational Tools for Analyzing Talk.* Hillsdale, NJ: Lawrence Erlbaum.

Maple, T. L., & Cone, S. G. (1981). Aged apes at the Yerkes Regional Primate Research Center. *Laboratory Primate Newsletter, 20,* 10–12.

Marler, P. (1990). Innate learning preferences: Signals for communication. *Developmental Psychobiology, 23(7),* 557–569.

Masataka, N. (1993). Effects of contingent and noncontingent maternal stimulation on the vocal behavior of three-to-four-month-old Japanese infants. *Journal of Child Language, 20,* 303–312.

McCarthy, D. (1954). Language development in children. In P. Mussen (Ed.), *Carmichael's manual of child psychology.* New York: Wiley.

Miles, H. L. (1983). Apes and language: The search for communicative competence. In J. deLuce & H. T. Wilder (Eds.), *Language in primates: Perspectives and implications.* New York: Springer-Verlag.

Nelson, K., & Lucariello, J. (1985). The development of meaning in first words. In M. Barrett (Ed.), *Children's single word speech.* Chichester, England: Wiley.

Papandropoulou, I., & Sinclair, H. (1974). What is a word? *Human Development, 17,* 241–258.

Patterson, F. G. P., & Cohn, R. H. (1990). Language acquisition by a lowland gorilla: Koko's first ten years of vocabulary development. *Word, 41,* 97–143.

Pellegrini, A. D., Brody, G. H., & Stoneman, Z. (1987). Children's conversational competence with their parents. *Discourse Processes, 10,* 93–106.

Pepperberg, I. M. (1991, Spring). Referential communication with an African grey parrot. *Harvard Graduate Society Newsletter,* 1–4.

Pepperberg, I. M. (1994) Vocal learning in grey parrots (psittacus erithacus): Effects of social interaction, reference, and context. *The Auk, 111,* 300–314.

Pinker, S. (1995). *The language instinct.* New York: Harper Perennial.

Premack, A. J. (1976). *Why chimps can read.* New York: Harper and Row.

Réger, Z., & Gleason, J. Berko. (1991). Romāni child-directed speech and children's language among Gypsies in Hungary. *Language in Society, 20,* 601–617.

Rumbaugh, D. M. (1977). *Language learning by a chimpanzee: The Lana project.* New York: Academic Press.

Rymer, R. (1993). Genie: An abused child's flight from silence. New York: Harper Collins.

Savage-Rumbaugh, E. S. (1990). Language acquisition in a nonhuman species: Implications for the innateness debate. *Developmental Psychobiology, 23(7),* 599–620.

Savage-Rumbaugh, E. S. (1993). Language learnability in man, ape, and dolphin. In H. L. Roitblat, L. M. Herman & P. E. Nachtigall (Eds.), *Language and communication: Comparative perspectives. Comparative cognition and neuroscience* (pp. 457–484). Hillsdale, NJ: Lawrence Erlbaum.

Savage-Rumbaugh, E. S., & Lewin, R. (1994). *Kanzi: The ape at the brink of the human mind.* New York: Wiley.

Shaywitz, B. A., Shaywitz, S. E., Pugh, K. R., Constable, R. T., Skudlarski, P., Fulbright, R. K., Bronen, R. A., Fletcher, J. M., Shankweiler, D. P., Katz, L. & Gore, J. C. (1995). Sex differences in the functional organization of the brain for language. *Nature, 6515,* 607–610.

Skinner, B. F. (1957). *Verbal behavior.* Englewood, NJ: Prentice-Hall.

Slobin, D. (1979). *Psycholinguistics* (2nd ed.). Glenview, IL: Scott, Foresman.

Snow, C. E. (1977). The development of conversation between mothers and babies. *Journal of Child Language, 4,* 1–22.

Snow, C. E. (1983). Literacy and language: Relationships during the preschool years. *Harvard Educational Review, 55,* 165–189.

Snow, C. E. (1990). The development of definitional skill. *Journal of Child Language, 17,* 697–710.

Snow, C. E., Perlmann, R. Y., Gleason, J. Berko, & Hooshyar, N. (1990). Developmental perspectives on politeness: Sources of children's knowledge. *Journal of Pragmatics, 14,* 289–305.

Stoel-Gammon, C., & Cooper, J. (1984). Patterns of early lexical and phonological development. *Journal of Child Language, 2,* 247–271.

Tager-Flusberg, H., & Sullivan, K. (1995). Attributing mental states to story characters: A comparison of narratives produced by autistic and mentally retarded individuals. *Applied Psycholinguistics, 16,* 241–256.

Terrace, H. S. (1980). *Nim: A chimpanzee who learned sign language.* New York: Knopf.

Werker, J. F., & Tees, R. C., (1984). Cross-language speech perception: Evidence for perceptual reorganization during the first year of life. *Infant Behavior and Development, 7,* 49–64.

Van Cantfort, T. E., & Rimpau, J. G. (1982). Sign language studies with children and chimpanzees. *Sign Language Studies, 34,* 15–72.

Vittorini, L. (1991). Untitled report. *The Fund for Animals, 24,* 1. New York: Publication of The Fund for Animals.

von Frisch, K. (1950). *Bees, their vision, chemical senses, and language.* Ithaca, NY: Cornell University Press.

Chapter Two

Communication Development in Infancy

Jacqueline Sachs, *University of Connecticut*

Introduction

In this chapter we will discuss communication development in the infancy period before the child begins to use words. Although this stage is **preverbal**, we will see that the infant is responsive to language, vocalizes in a variety of ways, and, usually toward the end of the first year, discovers the possibility of communication through vocalizations and gestures. Not too many years ago most descriptions of child language, while probably containing some information about babbling, would have really started at the point that the child said the first word. (That is, after all, the big event that gets noted in the baby book!) We know now that there are many aspects of communication in the first year of life that establish the foundation for later stages in the acquisition of language.

We have seen in the first chapter that there is a biological basis for language. At birth, the infant's brain and sensory systems are prepared for the task of acquiring a language. The infant can hear even before birth. Sounds generated outside the mother's abdomen are experienced inside the amniotic sac (Querleu & Renard, 1981), and infants are affected by what they have heard before birth. They have heard their mothers' voices best, and at birth already prefer their mothers' voices over those of strangers (DeCasper & Fifer, 1980). DeCasper and Spence (1986) also showed that newborn infants preferred the acoustic properties of a speech passage that their mothers had recited while pregnant to a passage they had not heard before, and Mehler et al. (1988) found that four-day-old infants who had been exposed to French could distinguish utterances in their native language from those of another language (perhaps on the basis of prosodic characteristics).

Many of the sounds that are used in speech (including those in languages to which the infant has not been exposed) are well discriminated by the young infant

(Aslin, Pisoni, & Jusczyk, 1983; Eimas, Miller, & Jusczyk, 1987; Eimas, Siqueland, Jusczyk, & Vigorito, 1971). Whether these discrimination abilities reflect special mechanisms for the processing of speech (Eimas, 1974) or are a characteristic of the mammalian auditory system (Kuhl, 1987) is as yet not completely resolved. However, even during the first year of life the infant's speech perception abilities are being shaped by the language she is hearing, so that the ability to discriminate sounds that are not used in the infant's language gradually disappear (Burnham, Earnshaw, & Clark, 1991; Werker & Tees, 1984). Although the infant will not show signs of beginning to comprehend the meaning of language until late in the first year, by that time she will normally have had a great deal of experience listening to speech. Table 2.1 shows the typical pattern of responses to sounds and speech in the first year of life.

At birth, the infant cries, producing the first of many signals that inform the caregiver about his needs. In the first year of life, the types of vocalizations that the infant can produce change dramatically. Table 2.2 shows the typical order of emergence of various types of vocalizations in the first year, with approximate ages. Although there are individual differences in the ages at which an infant achieves the stages of vocal development, the pattern appears to be the same across a wide variety of environmental and developmental conditions (Oller et al., 1994). Chapter 3 will provide more detail on sound production during this period as it relates to the development of the ability to produce speech sounds.

In terms of our focus in this chapter, the sounds made by infants can be viewed in terms of their role in the relationship between the infant and the caregiver. With

Table 2.1	Examples of the Typical Order of Emergence of Responses to Sounds and Speech in the First Year, with Approximate Ages
Newborn	Is startled by a loud noise
	Turns head to look in the direction of sound
	Is calmed by the sound of a voice
	Prefers mother's voice to a stranger's
	Discriminates many of the sounds used in speech
1–2 mos.	Smiles when spoken to
3–7 mos.	Responds differently to different intonations (e.g., friendly, angry)
8–12 mos.	Responds to name
	Responds to "no"
	Recognizes phrases from games (e.g., "Peekaboo," "How big is baby?")
	Recognizes words from routines (e.g., waves to "bye-bye")
	Recognizes some words

Table 2.2	Examples of the Typical Order of Emergence of Types of Nonword Vocalizations in the First Year, with Approximate Ages
Newborn	Cries
1–3 mos.	Makes cooing sounds in response to speech ("oo," "goo")
	Laughs
	Cries in different ways when hungry, angry, or hurt
	Makes more speechlike sounds in response to speech
4–6 mos.	Plays with some sounds, usually single syllables (e.g., "ba," "ga")
6–8 mos.	Babbles with duplicated sounds (e.g., "bababa")
	Attempts to imitate some sounds
8–12 mos.	Babbles with consonant or vowel changes (e.g., "badaga," "babu")
	Babbles with sentencelike intonation (expressive jargon/conversational babble)
	Produces protowords

that first cry begins an amazingly complex interactive process, the success of which depends both on the ability of the infant to signal messages clearly, and the ability of the caregiver to interpret those signals. While cries will alert the caregiver to the infant's physical needs, other vocalizations such as cooing, laughing, and babbling are a sign of the infant's inherent interest in social contact.

In recent years, there has been great interest in the caregiver–infant dyad. (We will use the term *caregiver* because, even though many studies have looked at mothers and their infants, other communicative partners, including older children, also play a role in the infant's development.) The infant seems helpless, and indeed is completely dependent on its caregivers. However, human infants have biologically given attributes and behaviors that draw caregivers to them. They are not simply passive recipients of stimulation, but instead are active interactional partners who are equipped to obtain the experiences that they need to develop. How the infant acts affects the subsequent behavior of the caregiver (Lewis & Rosenblum, 1974; Worobey, 1989), as has been shown in studies of various aspects of communication, such as eye contact. For example, it has been found that eye contact is very important to caregivers in establishing an affective bond with the infant. Selma Fraiberg (1974) discovered that parents of congenitally blind children often had difficulty in relating to their infants for this reason. One of the first indications of abnormality noticed by parents of autistic infants is that the children avert their eyes (Stern, 1971). In contrast, the normally interacting dyad engages in "gaze coupling" that very much resembles conversational turn-taking (Jaffe, Stern, & Perry, 1973).

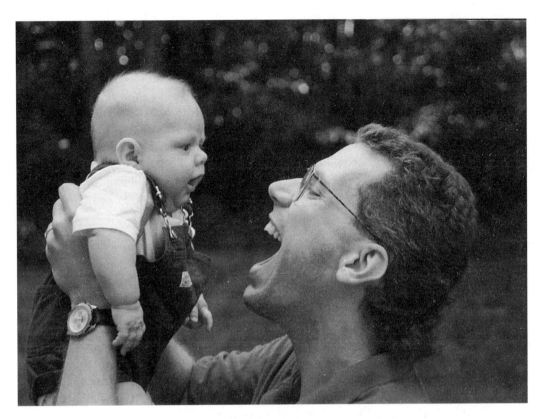

Gaze coupling in infancy is an important part of early communication development.

In vocal interaction, too, the caregiver is affected by the child's behavior. For example, in the course of carrying out research on young babies' vocalizations, Kathleen Bloom (1990) noticed that occasionally students and staff members who overheard the tapes made remarks like "That baby is really talking up a storm!" (p. 131). Thinking that perhaps the adults were responding to certain sorts of infant vocalizations, Bloom and Lo (1990) had adults rate videotapes of three-month-old babies who were making sounds that were more speechlike or less speechlike. The adults preferred the babies who produced sounds that were more like speech, rating them "cuddlier," "more fun," and generally more likable.

The cooing and babbling sounds that infants make also draw caregivers into "conversations" with them. By even three months of age, if an adult responds vocally to a baby's sounds, the baby in turn will begin to produce more speechlike sounds. Furthermore, babies learn to wait for the adult's response after they have vocalized. Thus, both the adult and the infant are constantly influencing one another in establishing conversation-like vocal interactions during a period well before the child uses words (Masataka, 1993).

The crying, cooing, and babbling of a young infant are already communicative in the sense that the infant is a member of a social species and the signals are salient to caregivers. However, in the latter part of the first year of life, the normally developing infant makes an important discovery that provides a transition to language—that one can intentionally make a signal (a vocalization or a gesture) and expect that it will have a specific effect on the caregiver. Thus signals begin to have meanings arising out of the shared experiences of the child and the caregiver. In the next section, we will look in more detail at what typically occurs in the emergence of **intentional communication**. After that, we will look at some aspects of the social context of the emergence of these behaviors. Although we have divided what the infant does and what caregivers do into two sections for organizational purposes, keep in mind that the behaviors of the infants and caregivers mutually affect one another.

The Expression of Communicative Intent before Speech

Characteristics of Intentional Communication

Although parents tend to view their infant's vocalizations as communicative and meaningful from as early as three months of age (Miller, 1988), there is little indication that the child deliberately behaves in a way that will obtain the adult's attention and help at that age (Bates, Camaioni, & Volterra, 1975).

Deciding whether any one instance of behavior is intentionally communicative or not is very difficult. Think, for example, of the behavior of a pet whose signals you interpret as meaning that the animal wants to be fed, let out, or petted. There has been much debate about the characteristics of intentional communication and the issue of whether the infant's behavior in the preverbal period is qualitatively different from that of other animals. Some researchers have suggested that, instead of using only one criterion for deciding whether a particular behavior is intentionally communicative, we use a set of criteria, applying them to the infant's entire behavior repertoire, to judge whether an infant is communicating with intentionality (Bakeman & Adamson, 1984; Bates, 1979; Bruner, 1973; Harding & Golinkoff, 1979; Scoville, 1983; Sugarman, 1984). The following are among the criteria that are often applied:

1. The child makes eye contact with the partner while gesturing or vocalizing, often alternating his gaze between an object and the partner.

2. The child's gestures and vocalizations become more consistent and ritualized. For example, a child named Annie used a gesture of opening and closing her hand rather than attempting to reach the object herself. The vocalization she used, "Eh eh," was one that she consistently used in situa-

tions in which she wanted something. Another child would probably have used a different sound in the same situation, because this sound is not copied from adult speech but rather is a communicative signal invented by the child.

3. The child may gesture or vocalize and wait for a response from the partner.

4. The child persists in attempting to communicate if he is not understood and sometimes even modifies his behavior to communicate more clearly.

When infants' behaviors are viewed in terms of such criteria, there does not appear to be a distinct boundary between behavior without communicative intent and intentional communication, but rather the child moves gradually toward an understanding of goals and the potential role of others in achieving them (Harding, 1983a, 1983b). In one study (Mosier & Rogoff, 1994), the mothers of infants ranging from six to thirteen months of age held or placed a desirable toy out of reach. Observers videotaped and scored the infants' gaze, gestures, and vocalizations for signs that the infant was trying to influence the mother, rather than simply attempting to get the toy or expressing frustration. In this situation, even six-month-old infants were judged as deliberately using their mothers to meet their goals, although this was the case in only 36 percent of the episodes.

Other investigators have usually reported that the first signs of intentional communication emerge between eight to ten months of age (e.g., Bates et al., 1975; Harding & Golinkoff, 1979). It is likely that even small differences in the situations observed or the criteria used to classify behaviors as intentional will affect judgments about the way these behaviors emerge, but certainly the change from inadvertent communicator to intentional communicator is a major one for both the child and that child's caregivers.

The Functions of Early Communicative Behaviors

Analyses of the functions of early communication stem from detailed observations of children's behaviors in various situations. For example, Michael Halliday (1975) studied his son Nigel's progress in attempting to communicate between nine and sixteen months, and found that several consistent nonword vocalizations seemed to convey meanings. Elizabeth Bates and her colleagues (Bates, 1979; Bates, Camaioni, & Volterra, 1975) reported on the gestures as well as preverbal vocalizations of the children they studied.

A number of different terms and systems of classification for early **communicative functions** have been proposed (e.g., Bruner, 1981; Chapman, 1981; Dore, 1974; Seibert & Hogan, 1982; Sugarman, 1984). Most systems distinguish at least among rejections, requests, and comments, often with further subcategories, as shown in Figure 2.1. The categories and examples of typical behavior cited in Figure 2.1 are:

Rejection
Request
 Request for social interaction
 Request for an object
 Request for action
Comment

Figure 2.1
Kinds of communicative functions that appear in the latter part of the first year of life

1. *Rejection.* Consistent gestures or vocalizations are used to terminate an interaction. For example, the child pushes away an offered object and vocalizes, or uses a gesture or vocalization to end an action. (You may also see rejections referred to by some authors as one form of **behavioral regulation,** that is, communication that serves to get the listener to do something or stop doing something.)

2. *Request:* Consistent gestures or vocalizations are used to get the partner to do something or to help the child achieve a goal. (Requests are also viewed as a form of behavioral regulation.)

 a. *Request for social interaction.* Behaviors are used to attract and maintain the partner's attention. For example, a child might use a vocalization as a greeting.

 b. *Request for an object.* For example, an abbreviated reaching gesture might be used to indicate desire for an object. In our earlier example, Annie obtained something she could not get herself by her vocalization and gesture. Later, this communicative function might be carried out by a word or phrase.

 c. *Request for action.* Consistent gestures or vocalizations are used to initiate an action by the listener. For example, the infant might lift her arms and use a vocalization when she wants to be picked up.

3. *Comment.* A consistent gesture or vocalization can be used to direct the partner's attention for the purpose of jointly noticing an object or event. For example, the infant might "show" an object to the caregiver by holding it out and vocalizing, or the infant might give an object to the caregiver. Pointing might be used not for the purpose of obtaining an object, but for directing the partner's attention to an object. (This function is also referred to as **joint attention.**)

All of these communicative functions are expressed by normally developing infants before they begin to use words (Wetherby, Cain, Yonclas, & Walker, 1988).

When children begin to talk at around twelve months of age, their words emerge within a rich framework of communicative functions that have been established toward the end of their first year of life.

The Forms of Early Communicative Behaviors

As an example of a communicative gesture, consider pointing. Pointing is unlike reaching for something—the index finger is extended while the other fingers are curled. The appropriate response to a point is to look in the direction indicated by the finger, not at the end of the finger itself. (When you have a chance, observe the response of a dog or cat to pointing.) Infants begin responding appropriately to points by others and pointing at objects or pictures themselves around ten months of age (Murphy, 1978; Zinober & Martlew, 1985). By twelve months, many infants point at an object and then shift their gaze to make eye contact with the listener (Bates, 1979; Masur, 1983).

The vocalizations used by children shortly before they begin learning conventional words have received much attention, because they form an interesting link between preverbal communication and speech. Intonation patterns can be used communicatively. For example, Halliday (1975), in the study mentioned above, observed his child using prelinguistic vocalizations with rising intonation contours for requests and falling contours for comments. Similar patterns have also been found in other children (Flax, Lahey, Harris, & Boothroyd, 1991; Menn, 1976).

Anne Carter (1979) studied a child named David over several months as he began to communicate intentionally, and noted that his preverbal vocalizations were initially quite variable in their pronunciation but were always linked with particular gestures. For example, several sounds similar to "ba" accompanied by waving hands seemed to signal that he did not want something, whereas sounds incorporating "mmm" accompanied by reaching meant that he did want it. Over time, the vocalizations became more phonetically stable and less tied to a particular action. Other investigators have also noticed that vocalizations and gestures are originally linked together, but become more independent over time (e.g., Greenfield & Smith, 1976).

Preverbal vocalizations that contain consistent sound patterns and are used in consistent situations, but are unique to the child rather than based on the adult language, are referred to as **protowords.** For example, an infant might start using the vocalization "lala" when he is rubbing his blanket against his cheek, and then use "lala" when he wants his blanket. Walburga von Raffler Engel (1973) noticed that her son used the sound "eee" when he wanted an object, but used "uuu" for disapproval. Other investigators studying children about eleven months of age have also found many vowel sounds consistently used with certain effects (Dore, Franklin, Miller, & Ramer, 1976). These investigators used the term **phonetically consistent form (PCF)** for protowords. Another term found for the same type of utterance is **vocable** (Ferguson, 1978; Werner & Kaplan, 1963).

How strong is the evidence that protowords are really inventions of the infant rather than sounds copied (perhaps from some chance association) from caregivers' speech? One body of research that supports this view involves detailed observations of communicative behaviors in young, profoundly deaf children. Most deaf children are born of hearing parents, and some hearing parents choose not to expose their deaf child to sign language in order to motivate the child to learn speech (following an oral approach to education of the deaf), while providing the child with a supportive social environment. Susan Goldin-Meadow and her colleagues (e.g., Goldin-Meadow, 1979; Goldin-Meadow & Morford, 1985) have found that these children develop spontaneous gestures that are not based on gestures used by the parents. Such early gestures, invented by the child, would be analogous to protowords invented by hearing children (though in the case of protowords, these idiosyncratic forms soon drop out when the child learns the conventional word to signal the meaning, whereas the deaf child's spontaneous gestures may develop into a richer communication system).

The Assessment of Communicative Intent

In order to assess whether a child is communicating intentionally, a method called **low-structured observation** is sometimes used (Coggins, Olswang, & Guthrie, 1987). The caregiver plays with the child in a natural way, and a trained observer scores the child's behavior during the session or from a videotape. For example, the observer would look for instances of commenting, as indicated by the child's pointing, showing, or giving objects (sometimes accompanied by consistent vocalizations).

One can structure the situation somewhat to increase the likelihood of observing requests by providing some items for play that are designed to serve as **communicative temptation tasks**—tasks that entice the child to produce requests (Casby & Cumpata, 1986; Dale, 1980; Snyder, 1984; Sugarman, 1978). For example, the child might be presented with an attractive toy inside a tightly covered plastic container. An infant who is not yet communicating intentionally might bang the container and fuss or cry in frustration, while another preverbal infant might hand the container to an adult, make eye contact, point to the toy and/or vocalize, and persist in such behaviors that seem to be directed toward the adult. (Another type of toy good for eliciting requests is a mechanical toy that has to be wound up by the adult.)

One can see how the child expresses rejection by having some less desirable toys along. If such a toy is given to the child while more desirable toys are in view, the child may potentially produce rejection gestures and/or vocalizations (Olswang, Bain, Dunn, & Cooper, 1983).

Cognitive Development and the Emergence of Intentional Communication

In the course of the first year of life, the infant's ability to form and use mental representations appears to change, as indicated by behavior in the face of various sorts of natural or experimental problem-solving situations. For instance, a young infant might reach out to grasp an attractive toy, but when the toy is moved out of her view, she stops reaching and appears not to remember her interest in the toy. Such behavior has been taken as an indication that the infant did not hold a mental image of the toy in mind that would provide the basis for a continued effort to obtain the toy.

The child's developing ability to solve various types of problems was studied in great detail by the Swiss psychologist Jean Piaget (e.g., Piaget, 1952). Piaget theorized that the infant is innately endowed with both certain reflexes and basic processes for learning from its interaction with objects in the environment, so that knowledge is constructed through a series of predictable stages in cognitive development. His descriptions of these stages in development have been very influential, and form the basis for much research about the relation between nonlinguistic thinking and language, as well as the basis for some clinical assessment of infants and children.

In the Piagetian framework, from birth until about eighteen to twenty-four months the infant is in the **sensorimotor stage,** and is beginning the process of learning how to think. The infant can experience objects through his senses and his actions with the objects, but does not yet have functional mental representations of them. However, there are changes in the infant's cognition within this period, two of which involve an understanding of the concept of object permanence and seeing the relation between activities and results of those activities (means-ends relations).

The concept of **object permanence** refers to the understanding that things exist even when we are not currently experiencing them. As in the example given above, if we see an object and then it is hidden from us, we continue to know that the object exists; we have a mental representation of it. However, for an infant in Stage 3 of the sensorimotor stage (at four to eight months), if an object is taken from view, the infant does not look for it. (The ages given are averages—some infants are faster or slower in cognitive development, but they will still pass through the same stages.) A Stage 4 infant (eight to 12 months) will look for an object if it disappears behind a screen, showing that the notion of object permanence is emerging. However, at this stage development is not complete. For example, if an object has been frequently hidden in one location, the infant will look there even after he sees it being hidden somewhere else.

The **means-ends concept** refers to the understanding that problems can be solved mentally, so that a goal can be attained by methods other than trial-and-error. At Stage 3, the infant may learn to make something happen again by repeating an activity that has led to the event, but does not seem to have a real sense of what could obtain the desired effect. During Stage 4, the infant begins to see the relation between actions and outcomes. For example, she may pull on a cloth to bring an object into reach. This is an example of primitive tool-using. At a later point the infant will experiment with actions to see what the result will be, and begin to be able to think ahead about what the result of an action might be. Also during this period, the infant will begin to anticipate what typically happens. For example, Piaget reported that at nine months his daughter would cry when someone stood up, because she had noticed that standing up was followed by leaving.

It has been found that the emergence of the ability to express communicative intent corresponds, at least temporally, with Stage 4 cognitive changes in the child such as those described above. For example, children do not begin to communicate intentionally until the time when they show, from other behaviors, that they understand something about means-ends relations. The child learns that it is possible to bring about changes through various means, and one of these means is to use another person to carry out one's goal. Thus the child is motivated to communicate to another person, rather than simply to attempt to achieve the goal himself (Bates, 1976; Harding & Golinkoff, 1979; Sugarman, 1978). [The interested reader should see Anisfeld (1984) for an extensive discussion of the relation between cognitive development and early language development.]

Although certain behaviors indicative of cognitive developments typically appear at the same time that certain language milestones do, we do not yet have convincing evidence that the cognitive changes are prerequisites for stages in language acquisition. Recent work in the field of cognitive development has shown that some abilities thought to develop at a certain time may be present much earlier. Jean Mandler (1990) states that "a good deal of evidence suggests that we have tended to confuse infants' motor incompetence with conceptual incompetence" (p. 240). For example, a series of studies on object permanence has involved a measure of infants' surprise rather than searching behavior and has demonstrated memory for objects even at three-and-one-half months (Baillargeon & DeVos, 1991).

The Social Context of the Preverbal Infant

Here we will look at some aspects of early communicative interaction between caregivers and preverbal infants. We will see that caregivers speak to infants in special ways, that they establish contexts for babies to take their turn at talk, and behave in other ways that may be supportive of the infant's attempts to communicate. We will not be able to describe all of the ways in which adults and infants communicate, but will concentrate on those aspects of communication that seem most closely related to later language development.

In describing the social context in which communication emerges, we are not arguing that social interaction causes the child to begin to communicate, or that adults teach their infants to communicate. Think, for example, of trying to be supportive of communicative development with your cat or dog. Clearly, one cannot teach a cat or a dog to react like a baby! The infant has the **biological capacity** for certain sorts of behaviors and abilities to develop. However, that biological capacity will not be realized without certain kinds of environmental supports. An important goal of research concerning the social context of communicative development is to find out what kinds of experiences are sufficient to allow development, and how variations in experiences ultimately affect the communicative abilities of the child (by *communicative abilities* we mean all aspects of language, including pragmatics).

The Sound of the Caregiver's Speech: "Listen to Me!"

Speech addressed to babies is typically quite unlike the speech directed to adults. We even have a name for it—**baby talk**. This term may initially merely bring to mind adult imitations of childlike speech ("Is ooo my tweetie-pie?") and special vocabulary words like *choo-choo* and *pottie,* along with strong denials that *you* would ever "use baby talk." However, as we will see here and in later chapters, there are actually many very interesting aspects of speech and language that are modified when we talk to infants and young children, and we make most of these modifications without even being aware of them. The primary difference between talk to babies and other speech is that "the **prosodic features** or 'music' appears to be more important than the words or 'lyrics'" (Stern & Wasserman, 1979, p. 3). Special intonation patterns with higher pitch, more variable pitch, and exaggerated stress have been found in baby talk in a variety of languages, including American English (e.g., Fernald & Simon, 1984; Garnica, 1977; Remick, 1976; Stern, Spieker, Barnett, & MacKain, 1983), Arabic (Ferguson, 1964), Marathi (Kelkar, 1964), Latvian (Ruke-Dravina, 1977), Mandarin Chinese (Grieser & Kuhl, 1988), and Japanese (Fernald et al., 1989).

Anne Fernald and her colleagues (Fernald, 1989; Fernald et al., 1989) have suggested that special intonation patterns may be a universal characteristic of baby talk. However, there are some differences in baby talk across cultures. Higher pitch and exaggerated intonation to infants were not found to be characteristic of rural African American families in North Carolina (Heath, 1983), Kaluli families in New Guinea (Schieffelin, 1979, 1990), and Quiche-Mayan families in Guatemala (Bernstein Ratner & Pye, 1984). Perhaps there are some general tendencies, such as using higher pitch, but these tendencies can be affected by other aspects of the way language is used in a particular culture. For example, Quiche-Mayan speakers use higher pitch as a sign of respect, and thus might find higher pitch socially inappropriate for use with a baby. Baby-talk speech modifications such as higher pitch may reflect social conventions that can vary from culture to culture (Ingram, 1995).

Next we will look in a little more detail at some of the possible reasons for the baby-talk characteristics that have been found in many cultures. (Keep in mind, though, that more research on diverse cultures and languages will be needed before we have a complete explanation.) Since certain prosodic features in speech to babies are common across many languages, it may be that these characteristics are used because they are especially appropriate. We can find out about babies' perceptual abilities and preferences by devising experiments in which they can "tell" us what they want to listen to. Infants cannot talk or press buttons, but they can turn their heads and control their eye movements, so a researcher might set up a situation in which a message plays only when the baby's head turns in a certain direction or when the eyes are fixated on a pattern, and measure the amount of time the baby thereby chooses to listen to one message or another. (A very important application of such techniques is for the testing of hearing in young infants.) A number of studies have shown that babies prefer baby-talk patterns (Fernald, 1985; Fernald & Kuhl, 1987; Sullivan & Horowitz, 1983; Werker & McLeod, 1989), even when only two days old (Cooper & Aslin, 1990), though it is not yet known exactly what characteristics of the baby talk lead to that preference (Cooper & Aslin, 1994).

If babies are naturally responsive to speech that has certain features, adults may use these characteristics because they discover or know intuitively that infants pay more attention to them when they do. By holding the infant's attention, the adult may help to cement the emotional bond between caregiver and child (Sachs, 1977). The attentive infant becomes quiet, faces the speaker, establishes eye contact, and responds to the adult. John Locke (1993, 1994) suggests that such communication provides the foundation for the child's entry into language learning: "Spoken language piggybacks on this open channel, taking advantage of mother–infant attachment by embedding new information in the same stream of cues" (Locke, 1994, p. 441). The voice will continue to carry information about emotional state, but the

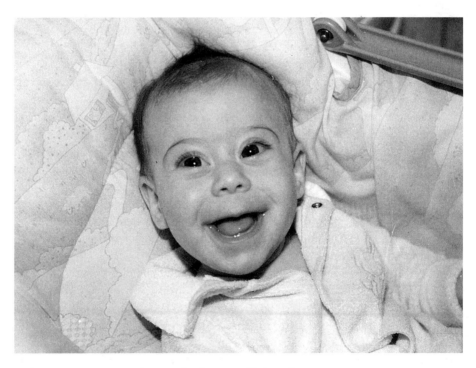

Infants are responsive to the prosodic features of baby talk.

child will eventually discover that it also consists of sounds, that these sounds create meaningful words, and that the words combine to convey even more complex messages. Children, of course, can learn language even if they are not in loving interactions, given their biologically based abilities, but adult-infant attachment may be involved in the optimal development of communication. For example, Cicchetti (1989) has reported significant language delays in maltreated toddlers. (For further discussion of the relation between affective development and communicative development, see Prizant & Wetherby, 1990.)

As the infant attends carefully to the caregiver's speech, opportunities arise for processing and comprehending some aspects of speech considerably before the emergence of the first word. For example, the exaggerated prosodic patterns of baby talk may help the infant become aware of the general communicative intent of a message, such as praising, prohibiting, playing, or comforting, before individual linguistic elements are understood (Fernald, 1989). Also, higher pitch and exaggerated stress tend to be used together on important parts of an utterance, such as the label for an object (Fernald & Mazzie, 1991), perhaps directing the infant's attention to those words.

The prosody of baby talk may even make it easier for infants to begin to segment larger units of speech. In one study, when preverbal seven- to nine-month-old babies heard samples of baby talk, they preferred to listen to messages in which the timing matched the natural clause structure of English rather than samples with altered clause structure. When the researchers played adult-directed speech to the babies, the babies did not discriminate between samples with natural and altered clause structure (Kemler-Nelson, Hirsh-Pasek, Jusczyk, & Wright-Cassidy, 1989).

Keep in mind that most studies have thus far been carried out in America with babies of urban, middle-class families. Since babies everywhere learn to speak, one must be cautious about concluding that some particular feature of baby talk is necessary (or even very useful) for babies. We do not know enough yet to tell caregivers how they *should* talk to babies. Research on language learning environments in a wide variety of cultures is needed (Blount, 1990), as is research to discover whether there are causal links between certain features of the linguistic environment and language learning.

The Conversational Nature of the Caregiver's Speech: "Talk to Me!"

Another characteristic of caregiver talk to infants is that it creates a two-way interpersonal engagement. Based on her observations of mothers interacting with babies in England, Catherine Snow (1977) argued that the mothers' primary goal in talking with their infants seemed to be to have a "conversation" with them. Even at an early stage when the adult knows that the infant does not yet understand language, the adult behaves as if the child's response is a turn in the conversation. First, here is a little "conversation" between a mother and her three-month-old daughter, Ann (p. 12).

Mother	Ann
	(smiles)
Oh what a nice little smile!	
Yes, isn't that nice?	
There.	
There's a nice little smile.	(burps)
What a nice wind as well!	
Yes, that's better, isn't it?	
Yes.	
Yes.	
Yes!	(vocalizes)
There's a nice noise.	

In this example, the mother spoke in short, simple utterances, although of course the three-month-old could not understand the content of the speech. The mother responded to whatever her infant did, commenting on the various nonverbal and vocal behaviors that occurred and incorporating them into the conversation. It is as if she allowed the infant's behaviors to stand for a turn in the interaction and treated the behavior as if it were intentional communication on the part of the infant.

Snow also noticed that the mothers devoted many of their utterances to attempting to elicit some kind of behavior from the infant, such as coos and smiles. In contrast to adult–adult conversations, where we often must try very hard to get our own turn, each mother seemed intent on giving her child a turn in the conversation. Many of the mothers' utterances were followed by pauses, providing the opportunity for responses from the infant, as in this example (Snow, 1977, p. 13):

Oh you are a funny little one, aren't you, hmm? Aren't you a funny little one? Hmm?

Although at three months the mother accepted almost any behavior on the part of the child as if it were an attempt to communicate, as the infants grew older, the mothers changed in what they accepted as a turn in the conversation. By seven months, when the babies had begun to be more active partners in the interactions, the mothers responded only to higher-quality vocalizations, such as a babbled sound, and not to sounds such as burps. Here is an example from a mutual babbling game, in which Ann's mother attempts to get her to imitate her vocalizations (Snow, 1977, p. 16).

Mother	Ann
Ghhhh ghhhh ghhhh ghhhh	
Grrrr grrrr grrrr grrr	(protest cry)
Oh you don't feel like it, do you?	aaaa aaaa aaaa
No I wasn't making that noise.	
I wasn't going *aaaa aaaa.*	aaaa aaaa
Yes, that's right.	

In this episode, the mother continued to make an attempt to structure the conversation so that Ann could take her turn, even though she was more demanding about what constituted a turn.

At twelve months the mothers' criteria for a turn had changed again, and they now attempted to interpret their children's vocalizations as words (Snow, 1977, p. 17).

Mother	Ann
	abaabaa
Baba. Yes that's you, what you are.	

Having seen that adults interact conversationally in certain ways with infants in the first year of life, we now consider the effect of this interaction.

The adult's linguistic behavior has an effect on the infant's behavior in the immediate situation. When mothers speak to three-month-old infants, the most common infant response is a vocalization (Lewis & Freedle, 1973). Furthermore, if the caregiver uses a conversational pattern of interaction, where the adult responds in a turn-taking manner to infant vocalizations, the type of sound a three-month-old baby will produce becomes more speechlike in response (Bloom, 1988).

It has also been suggested that the adult's interpretation of the infant's vocalizations may help the child get the idea that communication is possible (Harding, 1983a, 1983b). Adults interpret infants' behaviors as communicative long before the children have an intention to communicate. A two-month-old baby who is crying may be described by her mother as "wanting her diaper changed." The infant at this age is not actually intending a particular message but is crying because of discomfort. However, the fact that the mother accepts the cry as conveying a particular message creates the possibility for the child to begin to communicate different messages with different cries, and eventually perhaps notice the correspondence between the vocalizations and the effect it has on others.

What about long-term effects? We cannot yet conclude that any particular style of caregiver–infant interaction is necessary for language development. Children learn to talk with a wide range of linguistic experiences. For example, Elinor Ochs (1988) observed childrearing in Samoa and found that infants were typically not spoken to until they began to speak themselves (although, of course, they heard the speech going on around them). However, some research carried out on American families suggests that caregivers' language usage does at least affect the rate of language learning. For example, looking at the nine-to-eighteen-month period, Alison Clarke-Stewart (1973) found that the amount of talking that a mother did directly with her child (but not the amount of speech to others) was highly correlated with measures of the child's linguistic competence. This result would suggest that the overall quantity of speech that the child overhears is not so important for the rate of language development, but the quantity of direct adult-to-child talk is. Furthermore, infants whose mothers talk to them frequently using short utterances at nine months perform better on tests of receptive language abilities at eighteen months than do infants of less

vocally responsive mothers (Murray, Johnson, & Peters, 1990). Since lower socioeco-
nomic-status mothers within the United States talk less to their infants than do middle-class mothers (Richman et al., 1988), one important question for future research
is whether their less verbally interactive style, while sufficient for eventual language
acquisition, slows the acquisition process and ultimately puts their children at a disad-
vantage in terms of some aspects of broader communicative abilities. If that is the
case, it may be possible to improve children's communicative abilities by teaching
mothers to interact with them in a more responsive manner. (See Spiker, Ferguson &
Brooks-Gunn, 1993, for an example of one such early intervention project, and Bornstein, 1989, for a discussion of maternal responsiveness.)

Contexts for the Emergence of Object Reference: "Look at That!"

At about six months, infants begin to show a great interest in objects, perhaps reflecting both changes in their visual ability to scan their environment and their motor
ability to grasp and manipulate objects. While earlier the infant was entertained by
face-to-face social interactions, she now is drawn to investigate her surroundings. At
this point, the caregiver will usually change the strategy of interacting with the infant,
encouraging her to continue interpersonal interactions by jointly exploring objects
and their potential (Adamson & Bakeman, 1984). For example, one might see a playful interaction in which an older sibling dramatically wiggles a toy cow, saying "Look
at the *cow!* What does the cow say? The cow says 'mooooo.'" Caregivers label objects
(and also the actions or characteristics of objects) in play, in caregiving situations, in
looking at pictures in books, and in other social contexts of joint attention.

Research has shown, not surprisingly, that children whose mothers encourage
joint attention to objects and supply labels develop their vocabularies faster in the
early language acquisition period (e.g., Smith, Adamson, & Bakeman, 1988). Again,
one could ask whether we can at this point tell caregivers what they *should* do. For
example, it probably would not be a good idea to tell moms "Go around the house
and label everything in sight." Michael Tomasello and his colleagues (Tomasello,
1988; Tomasello & Farrar, 1986) have shown that words are most likely to be learned
if the caregiver focuses on what the *child* is interested in, providing a word at that
moment, rather than trying to direct the child's attention and actively teach the child
vocabulary.

Also, as in other areas we have considered, there can be cultural differences in
the pattern of joint attention involving objects. For instance, there are differences
between American mothers and Japanese mothers in the way they interact with
babies, even though both cultures are similar in paying a great deal of attention to
infants and children. American mothers encourage their young infants when they
look away from them with comments such as "Want to look around? There you go,"

whereas Japanese mothers discourage such looking away by saying things like "Say, look at me," and "What's wrong with you?" (Morikawa, Shand, & Kosawa, 1988, pp. 248–249). Also, American mothers tend to name objects when the infants attend to them, whereas Japanese mothers use those objects to engage their infants in social routines (Fernald & Morikawa, 1993). The authors of these reports noted that Americans tend to encourage independence in their children more than the Japanese do. Cultural values may begin to be transmitted by mother–infant interaction at a very early age, affecting subtle aspects of the mother–infant interaction.

In another observation in a different culture, it was found that !Kung San caregivers in Botswana were more likely to interact with an infant when he was not focusing on an object. If the infant was attending to an object, the caregivers did not try to join in that interaction in the way seen in many studies of American mothers (Bakeman, Adamson, Konner, & Barr, 1990). (For additional information on the development of joint attention during infancy and the implications of variations in the environment for our understanding of this aspect of development, see Adamson & Bakeman, 1991, and Adamson, 1991.)

Joint attention to objects accompanied by labeling by the caregiver of course provides an opportunity for the infant to begin to learn names for things. Studies of American infants have found that they generally comprehend many words, before they begin to say words themselves. For most children, the first evidence of word understanding occurs between eight and ten months. At eight months, more than half of a large sample of infants were reported to respond to three words that referred to people ("mommy," "daddy," and their own names), to some words from games and routines, such as "peekaboo," and to "bottle." By eleven months a child typically responded to about fifty words, including many names for common objects (Fenson et al., 1994).

Talk in Structured Situations: "Here's What We Say."

Jerome Bruner and his colleagues (e.g., Bruner, 1983; Ratner & Bruner, 1978) have described the possible development of early communication signals in structured situations. Bruner has used the term **format** (also called **scaffold**) to refer to such potential learning situations. One such context would be games that are often played with babies. Suppose that in playing a game such as riding "horsie" on daddy's knee, the infant is completely passive initially; he simply hears the words of the game and is moved about. Gradually, however, as the child learns what happens in the game, the father's expectations change. He comes to expect the infant to take a part in the game. Over time the father "raises the ante" so that more and more ritualized or conventional means of expression are demanded at various points in the game. Where the baby was jiggled, he now bounces up and down. Where the father said all of the words, perhaps a word is omitted to be filled in by a vocalization by the child. Eventually, within the game context, both father and child are truly communicating with each other. Such interactions may help the child get the idea that it is possible to communicate, and eventually know what is said in particular communicative situations.

Structured situations need not be games, of course. For example, Shirley Brice Heath (1983) has pointed out that even within American society there are speech communities in which games like pat-a-cake and peekaboo are not played. In some other cultures, play itself is not a central activity between mother and child (Ochs & Schieffelin, 1984; Schieffelin, 1990). Bruner (1982) has argued that though not all cultures will have play formats, they will have formats of some kind that facilitate the acquisition of language and culture. There may be certain things that are typically said in a feeding situation or when the infant is being dressed. Such routine events that occur frequently provide another way for the infant to begin noticing correspondences between sounds and meaning, initially leading to comprehension of words or phrases in the period just before the child will begin to say words.

The explanation of development that Bruner and other researchers who study the social context of language acquisition propose is similar to that of Lev Vygotsky (1978). Vygotsky was a Russian psychologist who criticized Piaget's theory that cognition developed primarily through the child's learning about the physical world. Vygotsky argued that infants are innately social beings and that one must include the role of the caregiver, who serves as a support for the child's acquisition of knowledge and skills, in any study of development. One concept that has influenced many contemporary researchers is the **zone of proximal development.** The zone of proximal development refers to the difference between what the child can do acting alone and what she can do when acting with the guidance of a caregiver. In terms of the emergence of intentional communication, the caregiver who is sensitive to an infant's current level of functioning cooperates with the child in a way that fosters growth. (For more information about Vygotsky's theory and its application to children's development, see Rogoff & Wertsch, 1984.)

A complete explanation of the emergence of intentional communication in the infant undoubtedly will have to consider the interaction of many factors, including at least the following: (1) the biological basis for language and changes that take place because of maturation of the central nervous system and peripheral structures, (2) the nonlinguistic cognitive development of the child, and (3) the types of experiences the child has had with caregivers. (See Hardy-Brown, 1983, for a discussion of the problems in disentangling maturational and experiential influences in development.) It is likely that there is both an inborn predisposition toward symbolic communication in the human infant and particular environmental experiences that interact with this predisposition to help bring about this important milestone in language development.

In this section on the social context of the infant, we have seen that caregivers typically speak in special ways to preverbal infants, behave as if infants are conversational partners well before they begin using language, and establish object and situationally focused contexts in which the correspondences between vocalizations and meaning can be discovered. Language normally has its beginning in a social communicative context, and patterns are established early that will continue to be used when a child's own speech emerges. There is some evidence that the specific characteristics of speech to prelinguistic infants play some role in their development. As one researcher in mother–infant communication put it, "The shared understandings which are built up between an infant and his familiars constitute the indispensable basic contexts for all his later interpersonal transactions, including the ones utilizing verbal language" (Bullowa, 1979, p. 12).

Summary

The first year of life—though the infant may not say a single word—is a very important period for communicative development. The infant is inherently social, responsive to caregivers, and draws caregivers into communicational interaction.

Perhaps one reason that the child enters so naturally into communication is that she is well equipped for perceiving speech sounds. Already at birth, infants appear to hear and discriminate speech sounds very well, and are thus well prepared to begin the process of acquiring language. Because infants can also discriminate sounds that they have not heard before, it seems likely that they are born with the ability to hear many sound categories that are used in different languages. Whether this perceptual ability has evolved in humans especially for speech, or reflects a general characteristic of the auditory system, is still unresolved.

In the first year of life, there are dramatic changes in the ability of the infant to produce sounds, reflecting physical growth, neurological maturation, and experiences with speech sounds. As the infant comes to control his articulatory structures, he progresses from simple cries to babbling to expressive jargon.

Finally, toward the end of the first year, children begin to behave in ways that seem intentionally communicative. They make gestures and vocalizations in a consistent and persistent manner to achieve goals. These early gestures and vocalizations are not learned from adults but are the child's own inventions. Through such means a child can express various communicative functions, such as rejecting, requesting, or commenting. It seems likely that the child achieves the milestone of intentional communication through maturation, changes in his underlying cognitive abilities, and through his experience with others.

Caregivers in many cultures talk to infants in special ways, typically with higher pitch and more variable intonation patterns. Such speech provides one source of affectionate stimulation for the young child, and babies are responsive to such stimulation. This attention-holding speech may also help the child to become aware of the linguistic function of vocalizations. The caregiver, in turn, accepts the child's responses to speech as early attempts at communication. Thus, the caregiver and infant can engage in "conversations" that provide a rich social context for the child's learning about language. Talking while jointly attending to objects and actions, and talking in frequently repeated situations, also exposes the infant to language in a way that may support language acquisition. Through research in this culture and others, we are coming to understand the ways in which parents and other caregivers naturally provide a setting for their children's acquisition of communicative competence.

At the end of the first year, the child is finally ready for the accomplishment that her caregivers view as the beginning of language—the first word—but the child has been preparing for that day from the very beginning.

Key Words

baby talk	object permanence
behavioral regulation	phonetically consistent form (PCF)
biological capacity	preverbal
communicative functions	prosodic features
communicative temptation tasks	protoword
format	scaffold
intentional communication	sensorimotor stage
joint attention	vocable
low-structured observation	zone of proximal development
means-ends concept	

Suggested Projects

1. Locate infants of several ages (for example, four, eight, and twelve months) and observe the speech of the parents or caregivers to them. It is preferable to make tape recordings, so that transcripts can be made and segments can be heard repeatedly. (It is difficult to listen for a number of features of speech at one time in a live observation session.) Choose particular features such as pitch, intonation patterns, rhythmic patterns, or repetition, and compare them in the tapes made at different ages. You might also want to compare caregivers—for example, observe both the mother and the father playing with the infant.

2. Locate babies at several ages, such as one, four, eight, and twelve months. Make tape recordings of the infants' vocalization in social settings with a caregiver. It is difficult to make transcriptions of infants' sounds even if you have had training in phonetic transcription. If you have had such training, attempt to transcribe some samples and see what problems you encounter. If you have not had such training, listen to the tapes and attempt to compare the sounds the babies make with the

sounds used in your language. Do you hear changes in the types of sounds from age to age?

3. Locate two babies, one about seven months and one about eleven months but not yet talking in words. Observe these babies interacting with caregivers in a relatively unstructured, playful situation. Take notes on each baby's vocalizations and behaviors, watching for signs of intentional communication (described on pages 44–45). Do you notice any differences between the two ages?

4. The notions of "communication," "intentionality" in communication, and "language" make very interesting topics for discussion. Think of various ways in which information is transmitted, within and across species. For example, wilted leaves on a plant might indicate to its caregiver that the plant needs water, and we often say things like "Ferns like to be kept moist," but we would not ordinarily think of the plant as communicating to us. If an animal or baby is shivering, we might infer that it is cold, without calling the shivering "communication." What counts as communicative behaviors? Is a cat meowing by its food bowl an example of intentional communication? Is an infant's vocable "eh eh" different from the cat's meow? How is using the word *blanket* different from using an invented form such as *lala*?

Suggested Readings

Anisfeld, M. (1984). *Language development from birth to three.* Hillsdale, NJ: Lawrence Erlbaum.

Bates, E. (1979). *The emergence of symbols: Cognition and communication in infancy.* New York: Academic Press.

Bruner, J. (1983). *Child's talk: Learning to use language.* New York: Norton.

Bullowa, M. (Ed.). (1979). *Before speech.* New York: Cambridge University Press.

Feagans, L., Garvey, C., & Golinkoff, R. (Eds.). (1983). *The origins and growth of communication.* Norwood, NJ: Ablex.

Foster, S. (1990). *The communicative competence of young children: a modular approach.* New York: Longman, Inc. (Particularly Chapters 2 and 3)

Golinkoff, R. (Ed.). (1983). *The transition from prelinguistic to linguistic communication.* Hillsdale, NJ: Lawrence Erlbaum.

Halliday, M. A. K. (1975). *Learning how to mean: Explorations in the development of language.* London: Edward Arnold.

Lock, A. (Ed.). (1978). *Action, gesture and symbol: The emergence of language.* New York: Academic Press.

Locke, J. L. (1993). *The child's path to spoken language.* Cambridge, MA: Harvard University Press.

Mandler, J. (1990). A new perspective on cognitive development in infancy. *American Scientist, 78,* 236–243.

Nadel, J., & Camaioni, L. (Eds.). (1993). *New perspectives in early communication development.* London: Routledge.

Schaffer, H. R. (1977). *Studies in mother–infant interaction.* New York: Academic Press.

References

Adamson, L. B. (1991). Variations in the early use of language. In L. T. Winegar & J. Valsiner (Eds.), *Children's development in social context: Vol. 1. Metatheory and Theory.* Hillsdale, NJ: Lawrence Erlbaum.

Adamson, L. B., & Bakeman, R. (1984). Mothers' communicative acts: Changes during infancy. *Infant Behavior and Development, 7,* 467–478.

Adamson, L. B., & Bakeman, R. (1991). The development of shared attention during infancy. In R. Vasta (Ed.), *Annals of Child Development* (Vol. 8). London: Kingsley.

Anisfeld, M. (1984). *Language development from birth to three.* Hillsdale, NJ: Lawrence Erlbaum.

Aslin, R. N., Pisoni, D. B., & Jusczyk, P. W. (1983). Auditory development and speech perception in infancy. In M. M. Haith & J. J. Campos (Eds.), *Handbook of child psychology: Vol. 2. Infancy and developmental psychobiology.* New York: Wiley.

Baillargeon, R. & DeVos, J. (1991). Object permanence in young infants: Further evidence. *Child Development, 62,* 1227–1246.

Bakeman, R., & Adamson, L. B. (1984). Coordinating attention to people and objects in mother–infant and peer–infant interaction. *Child Development, 55,* 1278–1289.

Bakeman, R., Adamson, L. B., Konner, M., & Barr, R. (1990). !Kung infancy: The social context of object exploration. *Child Development, 61,* 794–809.

Bates, E. (1976). *Language and context: The acquisition of pragmatics.* New York: Academic Press.

Bates, E. (1979). *The emergence of symbols: Cognition and communication in infancy.* New York: Academic Press.

Bates, E., Camaioni, L., & Volterra, V. (1975). The acquisition of performatives prior to speech. *Merrill-Palmer Quarterly, 21,* 205–224.

Bernstein Ratner, N., & Pye, C. (1984). Higher pitch in BT is not universal: Acoustic evidence from Quiche Mayan. *Journal of Child Language, 11,* 515–522.

Bloom, K. (1988). Quality of adult vocalizations affects the quality of infant vocalizations. *Journal of Child Language, 15,* 469–480.

Bloom, K. (1990). Selectivity and early infant vocalization. In J. R. Enns (Ed.), *The development of attention: Research and theory.* North-Holland: Elsevier Science Publishers.

Bloom, K., & Lo, E. (1990). Adult perceptions of vocalizing infants. *Infant Behavior and Development, 13,* 209–219.

Blount, B. (1990). Parental speech and language acquisition: An anthropological perspective. *Pre- and Peri-natal Psychology Journal, 4,* 319–337.

Blount, B., & Padgug, E. (1977). Prosodic, paralinguistic and interactional features in parent–child speech: English and Spanish. *Journal of Child Language, 4,* 67–86.

Bornstein, M. H. (1989). Between caretakers and their young: Two modes of interaction and their consequences for cognitive growth. In M. H. Bornstein & J. Bruner (Eds.), *Interaction in human development.* Hillsdale, NJ: Lawrence Erlbaum.

Bruner, J. (1973). Organization of early skilled action. *Child Development, 44,* 1–11.

Bruner, J. (1981). The social context of language acquisition. *Language and Communication, 1,* 155–178.

Bruner, J. (1982). The formats of language acquisition. *American Journal of Semiotics, 1,* 1–16.

Bruner, J. (1983). *Child's talk: Learning to use language.* New York: Norton.

Bullowa, M. (1979). Introduction: Prelinguistic communication: A field for scientific research. In M. Bullowa (Ed.), *Before speech.* New York: Cambridge University Press.

Burnham, D. K., Earnshaw, L. J., & Clark, J. E. (1991). Development of categorical identification of native and non-native bilabial stops: infants, children, and adults. *Journal of Child Language, 18,* 231–260.

Carter, A. (1979). Prespeech meaning relations: An outline of one infant's sensorimotor morpheme development. In P. Fletcher & M. Garman (Eds.), *Language acquisition.* Cambridge: Cambridge University Press.

Casby, M. W., & Cumpata, J. F. (1986). A protocol for the assessment of prelinguistic intentional communication. *Journal of Communication Disorders, 19,* 251–260.

Chapman, R. S. (1981). Exploring children's communicative intents. In J. Miller (Ed.), *Assessing Language Production in Children.* Austin, TX: PRO-ED.

Cicchetti, D. (1989). How research on child maltreatment has informed the study of child development: Perspectives from developmental psychopathology. In D. Cicchetti & V. Carlson (Eds.), *Child maltreatment. Theory and research on causes and consequences of child abuse and neglect.* New York: Cambridge University Press.

Clarke-Stewart, K. A. (1973). Interactions between mothers and their young children: Characteristics and consequences. *Monographs of the Society for Research in Child Development, 38* (Serial No. 153).

Coggins, T. E., Olswang, L. B., & Guthrie, J. (1987). Assessing communicative intents in young children: Low structured observation or elicitation tasks. *Journal of Speech and Hearing Disorders, 52,* 44–49.

Cooper, R. P., & Aslin, R. N. (1990). Preference for infant-directed speech in the first month after birth. *Child Development, 61,* 1584–1595.

Cooper, R. P., & Aslin, R. N. (1994). Developmental differences in infant attention to the spectral properties of infant-directed speech. *Child Development, 65,* 1663–1677.

Dale, P. (1980). Is early pragmatic development measurable? *Journal of Child Language, 7,* 1–12.

DeCasper, A. J., & Fifer, W. P. (1980). Of human bonding: Newborns prefer their mothers' voices. *Science, 208,* 1174–1176.

DeCasper, A., & Spence, M. (1986). Prenatal maternal speech influences newborns' perception of speech sounds. *Infant Behavior and Development, 9,* 133–150.

Dore, J. (1974). A pragmatic description of early language development. *Journal of Psycholinguistic Research, 3,* 343–350.

Dore, J., Franklin, M. B., Miller, R. T., & Ramer, A. L. H. (1976). Transitional phenomena in early language acquisition. *Journal of Child Language, 3,* 343–350.

Eimas, P. D. (1974). Auditory and linguistic processing of cues for place of articulation by infants. *Perception and Psychophysics, 16,* 513–521.

Eimas, P. D., Miller, J. L., & Jusczyk, P. (1987). On infant speech perception and the acquisition of language. In S. Harnad (Ed.), *Categorical perception.* Cambridge: Cambridge University Press.

Eimas, P. D., Siqueland, E. R., Jusczyk, P., & Vigorito, J. (1971). Speech perception in infants. *Science, 171,* 303–306.

Fenson, L., Dale, P. S., Reznick, J. S., Bates, E., Thal, D. J., & Pethick, S. J. (1994). Variability in early communicative development. *Monographs of the Society for Research in Child Development, 59* (Serial No. 242).

Ferguson, C. A. (1964). Baby talk in six languages. *American Anthropologist, 66,* 103–114.

Ferguson, C. A. (1978). Learning to pronounce: The earliest stages of phonological development in the child. In F. D. Minifie & L. L. Lloyd (Eds.), *Communication and cognitive abilities—Early behavioral assessment.* Baltimore: University Park Press.

Fernald, A. (1985). Four-month-old infants prefer to listen to motherese. *Infant Behavior and Development, 8,* 181–195.

Fernald, A. (1989). Intonation and communicative intent in mothers' speech to infants: Is the melody the message? *Child Development, 60,* 1497–1510.

Fernald, A., & Kuhl, P. K. (1987). Acoustic determinants of infant preference for motherese speech. *Infant Behavior and Development, 10,* 279–293.

Fernald, A., & Mazzie, C. (1991). Pitch-marking of new and old information in mothers' speech. Paper presented at a meeting of the Society for Research in Child Development.

Fernald, A., & Morikawa, H. (1993). Common themes and cultural variation in Japanese and American mothers' speech to infants. *Child Development, 64,* 637–656.

Fernald, A., & Simon, T. (1984). Expanded intonation contours in mothers' speech to newborns. *Developmental Psychology, 20,* 104–113.

Fernald, A., Taeschner, T., Dunn, J., Papousek, M., de Boysson-Bardies, B., & Fukui, I. (1989). A cross-language study of prosodic modifications in mothers' and fathers' speech to pre-verbal infants. *Journal of Child Language, 16,* 477–501.

Flax, J., Lahey, M., Harris, K., & Boothroyd, A. (1991). Relations between prosodic variables and communicative functions. *Journal of Child Language, 18,* 3–19.

Fraiberg, S. (1974). Blind infants and their mothers: An examination of the sign system. In M. Lewis & L. A. Rosenblum (Eds.), *The effect of the infant on its caregiver.* New York: Wiley.

Garnica, O. (1977). Some prosodic and paralinguistic features of speech to young children. In C. Snow & C. A. Ferguson (Eds.), *Talking to children.* New York: Cambridge University Press.

Goldin-Meadow, S. (1979). Structure in a manual communication system developed without a conventional language model: Language without a helping hand. In H. Whitaker & H. A. Whitaker (Eds.), *Studies in neurolinguistics* (Vol. 4). New York: Academic Press.

Goldin-Meadow, S., & Morford, M. (1985). Gesture in early child language: Studies of deaf and hearing children. *Merrill-Palmer Quarterly, 31,* 145–176.

Greenfield, P., & Smith, J. (1976). *The structure of communication in early language development.* New York: Academic Press.

Grieser, D. L., & Kuhl, P. K. (1988). Maternal speech to infants in a tonal language: Support for universal prosodic features in motherese. *Developmental Psychology, 24,* 14–20.

Halliday, M. A. K. (1975). *Learning how to mean: Explorations in the development of language.* London: Edward Arnold.

Harding, C. G. (1983a). Acting with intention: A framework for examining the development of intention. In L. Feagans, C. Garvey, & R. Golinkoff (Eds.), *The origins and growth of communication.* Norwood, NJ: Ablex.

Harding, C. G. (1983b). Setting the stage for language acquisition: Communication development in the first year. In R. M. Golinkoff (Ed.), *The transition from prelinguistic to linguistic communication.* Hillsdale, NJ: Lawrence Erlbaum.

Harding, C. G., & Golinkoff, R. M. (1979). The origins of intentional vocalizations in prelinguistic infants. *Child Development, 50,* 338–340.

Hardy-Brown, K. (1983). Universals and individual differences: Disentangling two approaches to the study of language acquisition. *Developmental Psychology, 19,* 610–624.

Heath, S. B. (1983). *Ways with words: Language, life and work in communities and classrooms.* Cambridge, UK: Cambridge University Press.

Ingram, D. (1995). The cultural basis of prosodic modifications to infants and children: A response to Fernald's universalist theory. *Journal of Child Language, 22,* 223–233.

Jaffe, J., Stern, D., & Perry, C. (1973). "Conversational" coupling of gaze behavior in prelinguistic human development. *Journal of Psycholinguistic Research, 2,* 321–330.

Kelkar, A. (1964). Marathi baby talk. *Word, 20,* 40–54.

Kemler-Nelson, D. G., Hirsh-Pasek, K., Jusczyk, P. W, & Wright-Cassidy, K. (1989). How the prosodic cues in motherese might assist language learning. *Journal of Child Language, 16,* 53–68.

Kuhl, P. (1987). Perception of speech and sound in early infancy. In P. Salapatek & L. Cohen (Eds.), *Handbook of infant perception: Vol. 2. From perception to cognition.* New York: Academic Press.

Lewis, M., & Freedle, R. (1973). Mother–infant dyad: The cradle of meaning. In P. Pliner, L. Krames, & T. Alloway (Eds.), *Communication and affect, language and thought.* New York: Academic Press.

Lewis, M., & Rosenblum, L. A. (Eds.). (1974). *The effect of the infant on its caregiver.* New York: Wiley.

Locke, J. L. (1993). *The child's path to spoken language.* Cambridge, MA: Harvard University Press.

Locke, J. L. (1994). Phases in the child's development of language. *American Scientist, 82,* 436–445.

Mandler, J. (1990). A new perspective on cognitive development in infancy. *American Scientist, 78,* 236–243.

Masataka, N. (1993). Effects of contingent and noncontigent maternal stimulation on the vocal behavior of three- to four-month-old Japanese infants. *Journal of Child Language, 20,* 303–312.

Masur, E. F. (1983). Gestural development, dual-directional signaling and the transition to words. *Journal of Psycholinguistic Research, 12,* 93–109.

Mehler, J., Jusczyk, P., Lambertz, G., Halsted, N., Bertoncini, J., & Amiel-Tison, C. (1988). A precursor of language acquisition in young infants. *Cognition, 29,* 143–178.

Menn, L. (1976). *Pattern, control, and contrast in beginning speech: A case study in the acquisition of word form and function.* Unpublished doctoral dissertation, University of Illinois.

Miller, C. L. (1988). Parents' perceptions and attributions of infant vocal behaviour and development. *First Language, 8,* 125–142.

Morikawa, H., Shand, N., & Kosawa, Y. (1988). Maternal speech to prelingual infants in Japan and the United States: Relationships among functions, forms and referents. *Journal of Child Language, 15,* 237–256.

Mosier, C. E., & Rogoff, B. (1994). Infants' instrumental use of their mothers to achieve their goals. *Child Development, 65,* 70–79.

Murphy, C. M. (1978). Pointing in the context of a shared activity. *Child Development, 49,* 371–380.

Murray, A. D., Johnson, J., & Peters, J. (1990). Fine-tuning of utterance length to preverbal infants: Effects on later language development. *Journal of Child Language, 17,* 511–526.

Ochs, E. (1988). *Culture and language development. Language acquisition and language socialization in a Samoan village.* New York: Cambridge University Press.

Ochs, E., & Schieffelin, B. (1984). Language acquisition and socialization: Three developmental stories and their implications. In R. Shweder & R. LeVine (Eds.), *Culture theory: Essays on mind, self and emotion.* New York: Cambridge University Press.

Oller, D. K., Eilers, R. E., Steffens, M. L., Lynch, M. P., & Urbano, R. (1994). Speech-like vocalizations in infancy: An evaluation of potential risk factors. *Journal of Child Language, 21,* 33–58.

Olswang, L., Bain, B., Dunn, C., & Cooper, J. (1983). The effects of stimulus variation on lexical learning. *Journal of Speech and Hearing Disorders, 48,* 192–201.

Piaget, J. (1952). *The origins of intelligence in children.* New York: International Universities Press.

Prizant, B. M., & Wetherby, A. M. (1990). Toward an integrated view of early language and communicative development and socioemotional development. *Topics in Language Disorders, 10,* 1–16.

Querleu, D., & Renard, K. (1981). Les perceptions auditives du foetus humain. *Medicine et Hygiene, 39,* 2102–2110.

Ratner, N. K., & Bruner, J. S. (1978). Games, social exchange and the acquisition of language. *Journal of Child Language, 5,* 391–401.

Remick, H. (1976). Maternal speech to children during language acquisition. In W. von Raffler Engel & Y. Lebrun (Eds.), *Baby talk and infant speech.* Amsterdam: Swets and Zeitlinger.

Richman, A., LeVine, R., New, R., Howrigan, G., Wells-Nystrom, B., & LeVine, S. (1988). Maternal behavior to infants in five cultures. In R. LeVine, P. Miller, & M. West (Eds.), Parental behavior in diverse societies. *New Directions in Child Development* (No. 40), 81–98.

Rogoff, B., & Wertsch, J. V. (1984). *Children's learning in the "zone of proximal development."* San Francisco: Jossey-Bass.

Ruke-Dravina, V. (1977). Modifications of speech addressed to young children in Latvian. In C. Snow & C. A. Ferguson (Eds.), *Talking to children.* New York: Cambridge University Press.

Sachs, J. (1977). The adaptive significance of linguistic input to prelinguistic infants. In C. Snow & C. A. Ferguson (Eds.), *Talking to children.* New York: Cambridge University Press.

Schieffelin, B. B. (1979). Getting it together: An ethnographic approach to the study of the development of communicative competence. In E. Ochs & B. B. Schieffelin (Eds.), *Developmental pragmatics.* New York: Academic Press.

Schieffelin, B. B. (1990). *The give and take of everyday life: Language socialization of Kaluli children.* Cambridge, UK: Cambridge University Press.

Scoville, R. (1983). Development of the intention to communicate: The eye of the beholder. In L. Feagans, C. Garvey, & R. Golinkoff (Eds.), *The origins and growth of communication.* Norwood, NJ: Ablex.

Seibert, J., & Hogan, A. (1982). *Procedures manual for the early social-communication scales.* Miami: University of Miami.

Smith, C. B., Adamson, L. B., & Bakeman, R. (1988). Interactional predictors of early language. *First Language, 8,* 143–156.

Snow, C. (1977). The development of conversation between mothers and babies. *Journal of Child Language, 4,* 1–22.

Snyder, L. (1984). Communicative and cognitive abilities and disabilities in the sensorimotor period. *Merrill-Palmer Quarterly, 24,* 161–180.

Spiker, D., Ferguson, J., & Brooks-Gunn, J. (1993). Enhancing maternal interactive behavior and child social competence in low birth weight, premature infants. *Child Development, 64,* 754–768.

Stern, D. N. (1971). A micro-analysis of mother–infant interaction. *Journal of the American Academy of Child Psychiatry, 10,* 501–517.

Stern, D. N., Spieker, S., Barnett, R., & MacKain, K. (1983). The prosody of maternal speech: Infant age and context related changes. *Journal of Child Language, 10,* 1–15.

Stern, D. N., & Wasserman, G. A. (1979). Maternal language to infants. Paper presented at a meeting of the Society for Research in Child Development.

Sugarman, S. (1978). Some organizational aspects of pre-verbal communication. In I. Markova (Ed.), *The social context of language.* London: Wiley.

Sugarman, S. (1984). The development of preverbal communication. In R. Schiefelbusch & J. Pickar (Eds.), *The acquisition of communicative competence.* Baltimore: University Park Press.

Sullivan, J. W., & Horowitz, F. D. (1983). The effects of intonation on infant attention: The role of the rising intonation contour. *Journal of Child Language, 10,* 521–534.

Tomasello, M. (1988). The role of joint attentional processes in early language development. *Language Sciences, 10,* 69–88.

Tomasello, M., & Farrar, M. J. (1986). Joint attention and early language. *Child Development, 57,* 1454–1463.

von Raffler Engel, W. (1973). The development from sound to phoneme in child language. In C. A. Ferguson & D. Slobin (Eds.), *Studies of child language development.* New York: Holt, Rinehart & Winston.

Vygotsky, L. (1978). *Mind in society: The development of higher psychological processes.* Cambridge, MA: Harvard University Press.

Werker, J. F., & Tees, R. C. (1984). Cross-language speech perception: Evidence for perceptual reorganization during the first year of life. *Infant Behavior and Development, 7,* 49–64.

Werker, J., & McLeod, P. J. (1989). Infant preference for both male and female infant-directed talk: A developmental study of attentional and affective responsiveness. *Canadian Journal of Psychology, 43,* 230–246.

Werner, H., & Kaplan, B. (1963). *Symbol formation.* New York: Wiley.

Wetherby, A., Cain, D., Yonclas, D., & Walker, V. (1988). Analysis of intentional communication of normal children from the prelinguistic to the multi-word stage. *Journal of Speech and Hearing Research, 31,* 240–252.

Worobey, J. (1989). Mother–infant interaction: Protocommunication in the developing dyad. In J. F. Nussbaum (Ed.), *Life-span communication: Normative processes.* Hillsdale, NJ: Lawrence Erlbaum.

Zinober, B., & Martlew, M. (1985). Developmental changes in four types of gesture in relation to acts and vocalization from 10 to 21 months. *British Journal of Developmental Psychology, 3,* 293–306.

Chapter Three

Phonological Development: Learning Sounds and Sound Patterns

Carol Stoel-Gammon, *University of Washington*
Lise Menn, *University of Colorado*

Introduction

Everyone knows that children's early attempts at words may sound quite different from adult pronunciations. We are familiar with some typical early word pronunciations, and we feel that they are somehow simplified (though it is not obvious why *wed* should be easier to say than *red,* or *tat* easier than *cat*). However, there are many other types of early pronunciations that adults are generally not aware of, such as *sore* for *store,* or *gig* for *pig.* Theories of phonetic and phonological development must explain why both the familiar and the less common early word forms may appear.

In this chapter, we describe and explain children's pronunciation in the first year or so after they begin to use words; then we look at some research on the later aspects of phonological development. To begin with, however, we must study the speech sounds themselves and see what is involved in learning to produce them, for adults tend to take this incredible skill for granted.

English Speech Sounds and Sound Patterns

Our first step is to establish a way of referring to speech sounds that will avoid the ambiguities of the English spelling system. Descriptions of sounds in terms like *hard* and *soft, long* and *short* rapidly become too cumbersome. The ambiguity of the letter *c* is only one kind of mismatch between English spelling and English speech sounds. Another kind arises when English uses two letters to spell a unitary sound, like *sh*. A third comes about because there are multiple ways of spelling almost any given sound—for example, the *f* in *fat* can also be spelled *ff, ph,* and even *gh* (as in *cough*). Such mismatches make it misleading even to think of spoken words as being composed of letters; that term is therefore reserved for written words. This chapter, like much of the literature on language development and linguistics, will refer to speech sounds or to segments; technical terms for the elements that compose spoken words will be defined. For written reference to speech sounds, we will use a system called the International Phonetic Alphabet (IPA). The symbols presented in Table 3.1 represent the basic speech sounds of general American English.

Phonetics: The Production and Description of Speech Sounds

The sounds of any language are cross-classified in a web of similarities and differences of pronunciation, and understanding the reasons for these similarities and differences is the key to understanding young children's speech patterns. One of these classifications, the division into vowel and consonant, is part of school grammar, and many of the others are reasonably straightforward. For example, the sounds [p], [b], and [m] have in common the property that they are all produced with the lips closed.

Table 3.1   **Phoneme Symbols for Speech Sounds of General American English**

Symbol	Example	Symbol	Example	Symbol	Example	Symbol	Example	Symbol	Example
		Vowels				*Consonants*			
/i/	b*ea*d	/ʊ/	p*u*t	/p/	*p*ill	/f/	*f*ie	/h/	*h*i
/ɪ/	b*i*d	/uw/	b*oo*t	/t/	*t*ill	/θ/	*th*igh	/m/	ra*m*
/ej/	b*ai*t	/ʌ/	p*u*tt	/k/	*k*ill	/s/	*s*igh	/n/	ra*n*
/ɛ/	b*e*t	/ɝ/	b*ir*d	/b/	*b*ill	/ʃ/	*sh*y	/ŋ/	ra*ng*
/æ/	b*a*t	/aj/	b*i*te	/d/	*d*ill	/v/	*v*at	/l/	*l*ed
/a/	t*o*t	/æw/	b*ou*t	/g/	*g*ill	/ð/	*th*at	/r/	*r*ed
/ɔ/	t*au*ght	/ɔj/	b*oy*	/tʃ/	*ch*ill	/z/	*C*aesar	/j/	*y*et
/ow/	t*o*te	/ə/	*a*bout[1]	/dʒ/	*J*ill	/ʒ/	sei*z*ure	/w/	*w*et

[1]This vowel occurs in unstressed syllables only.

Descriptive Features: Classifying Sounds by How They Are Produced

Descriptive features, as the name implies, are used to describe and classify each speech sound in terms of the *source* of the sound in the vocal tract and the *shape* of the vocal tract during sound production. Speech sounds are created as air passes through the vocal tract (larynx, pharynx, mouth, and nose); the shape is varied by moving the lips, tongue, and lower jaw. The sound waves that we hear are set in motion either by vocal cord vibration or by the friction of airstream turbulence. (Kissing and clucking mouth noises are examples of other oral sound sources.) Although they are not incorporated into English words, some other languages, such as Zulu and Xhosa (spoken in South Africa), do use such sound sources for their "click" consonants.

If the source of a speech sound is partly or entirely vocal cord vibration, it is called a **voiced** sound. It is easy to tell whether a sound is voiced: voiced sounds can be hummed or sung, at least for a fraction of a second, but unvoiced sounds cannot, since it takes vocal cord vibration to produce a singing tone.

Turbulence (airstream friction) has the sound of air hissing slowly out of a tire; we hear it in speech sounds like [s] and [f]. Turbulence occurs when air is forced through a narrow opening. In the vocal tract, the narrow opening is usually made by bringing the lower articulators (lower lip, teeth, and tongue) close to the upper articulators (upper lip, teeth, and roof of the mouth). The sound produced by the vocal cords or airstream friction takes on different qualities depending on the exact position of the lips, jaws, and tongue; thus, [f] sounds different from [s] even though both have friction as their source, and [a] sounds different from [i] even though both have the vibration of vocal cords as their source. The study of how the shape of the vocal tract gives sounds their distinct identities is **acoustic phonetics.**

The Major Sound Classes

Vowel sounds are made with the vocal tract relatively unobstructed so that air moves through it smoothly; vocal cord vibration is the only sound source. Different vowel sounds result from varying the positions of the articulators: how wide the jaw opening is, whether the bulk of the tongue is held toward the front or the back of the mouth, and whether the lips are pursed, relaxed, or pulled out into a smile position. (Photographers ask their subjects to say "cheese" because the sounds of this word shape the mouth into a smile.)

Consonant sounds are made with a more constricted vocal tract and are classified on the basis of three aspects of their production: *place of articulation* (that is, which articulators are involved), *manner of articulation* (how the speech sound is produced), and *voicing* (presence or absence of vocal cord vibration during production). Table 3.2 provides a classification of the consonants of American English using these

Table 3.2 **Classification of Consonants**

Place	Bilabial	Labiodental	Interdental	Alveolar	Palatal	Velar	Glottal
Manner							
Stop	p b			t d		k g	
Fricative		f v	θ ð	s z	ʃ ʒ		h
Affricate					tʃ dʒ		
Nasal	m			n		ŋ	
Liquid				l	r		
Glide	w				j		

three features. We have already mentioned some of the consonants whose sound source is airstream friction produced in the mouth; these are called **fricatives**. Besides [f] and [s], the class of fricatives includes [θ] (as in *thigh*) and [ʃ] (as in *shy*); these four fricatives are produced without vocal cord vibration and are thus **unvoiced fricatives**. English has four other speech sounds made with turbulence in the mouth—[v], [z], [ð] (as in *the*) and [ʒ] (the second consonant of the word *seizure*); these four are produced with vocal cord vibration in addition to friction, and are subclassified as **voiced** fricatives. Another friction sound is [h], a voiceless consonant usually produced with friction in the glottis (the space between the vocal cords); [h] is called a **glottal fricative**.

The consonants made with the tightest vocal tract constriction are the stops, which are produced with upper and lower articulators pressed together so tightly that no air can escape from the mouth. The class of **unvoiced stops** is composed of [p], [t], and [k]; the set of **voiced stops** includes [b], [d], and [g]. Consonants classified as **affricates** begin like a stop and end like a fricative; [tʃ], the first sound of *chill*, is a **voiceless affricate**; [dʒ], as in *Jill*, is a **voiced affricate**. Together, stop, fricative and affricate consonants are referred to as **obstruents** because they fully or partially obstruct the oral airflow.

During normal breathing, air from the lungs exits from the nose. In the production of most speech sounds, however, including the ones already described, the passage from the pharynx to the nose is closed off by raising the **velum** (soft palate), a soft tissue extension of the roof of the mouth (hard palate), as shown in Figure 3.1. However, three speech sounds of English, the **nasal stops** [m], [n], and [ŋ], are made with the velum lowered so that air can escape through the nose; you can check that it does so by humming [m] or [n]. English speakers are often unaware of the third nasal stop listed here, the [ŋ], partly because it does not have its own symbol in the alphabet. It is the sound spelled *n* in *finger* and in *sink* (verify for yourself that this sound is not an [n]);

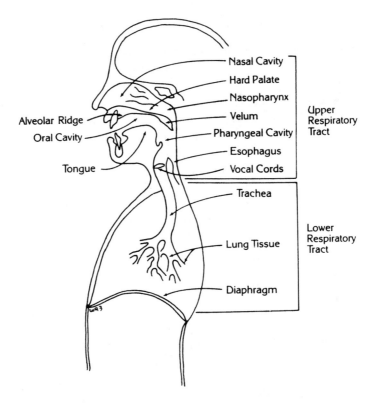

Figure 3.1
The vocal tract

it is also the final sound in words that end with the letters *ng,* such as *sing.* In most varieties of English, there is no [g] pronounced at the end of these words.

The **glides** [j] and [w] are made with a little more vocal tract constriction than the vowels and are often called **semivowels.** Traditional English grammar groups the glides with the consonants, but phonologically they are usually considered as lying in between the true consonants and the vowels.

The **liquids** [r] and [l] are made with a little more constriction in the vocal tract than the glides, but still not enough to cause friction; they also have characteristics intermediate between vowels and obstruent consonants. One important vowel-like characteristic is the role that liquids can play in syllable structure; we usually think of a syllable as having to contain a vowel, but there are syllables in which a liquid is used as if it were a vowel. The second syllable of *legal* is spelled with an *a,* but what we say is /li-gl/ or /lig-l/; and in most varieties of American English, the noun *record* is /rɛ-krd/. The nasal sounds also have this capacity to serve in place of vowels in certain syllables: consider *random* /ræn-dm/ and *season* /si-zn/.

The Shape of the Vocal Tract: Position of Articulation

The point at which the upper and lower articulators (upper lip, upper teeth, roof of the mouth; lower lip, lower teeth, tongue) touch or approach each other most closely is usually called the place of articulation. As mentioned, the sounds [p], [b], and [m] are all produced with the same mouth position; the lips are closed. They, therefore, are labeled as **labial** (or *bilabial*). Moving from the lips toward the back of the mouth, the other positions usually used in describing English sounds are:

> **Labiodental.** This term is used to describe sounds articulated with the lower lip resting lightly against the upper teeth. A slight space is left between the lip and teeth for the air to escape. This is the position of articulation for [f] and [v].
>
> **Interdental.** This term describes sounds made with the tongue lightly touching the upper teeth, perhaps projecting out slightly beyond them. This is the position of articulation for [θ], as in *thigh,* and [ð], as in *thy.*
>
> **Alveolar.** This term refers to sounds made with the tongue in contact with the alveolar ridge. This is the point behind the upper teeth where the front of the tongue makes contact in producing [t], [d], or [n] in English. The [s] and [z] sounds are also alveolar; they are made with the tongue in essentially the same position as [t], [d], and [n], but not quite in contact with the alveolar ridge since [s] and [z] are fricatives. The sound [l] (at the beginnings of syllables) is also made with the front of the tongue touching the alveolar ridge, but [l] is not a stop; in making [l], air escapes from the mouth by passing out between the side of the tongue and the upper teeth.
>
> **Palatal.** This term is used to refer to sounds articulated with the tongue near or contacting the hard palate and/or the slope leading up to it from the alveolar ridge. The tongue makes contact in the palatal area for production of the fricatives [ʃ] and [ʒ] and the affricates [tʃ] and [dʒ]. The tongue is positioned near the hard palate for the glide [j] and the liquid [r].
>
> **Velar.** This term refers to sounds made when the back of the tongue touches the velum, as in the production of [k], [g], or [ŋ].
>
> **Glottal.** This term refers to sounds produced in the area of the glottis, and denotes the place of articulation of the fricative [h].

English has no velar fricatives, but many other languages do, including German and Russian. There are many other descriptive features; some additional ones are needed for describing English, and even more are needed for sounds found in other languages of the world, and in children's babbling and speech. We will not attempt a larger catalog here but will define additional features as we need them.[1]

---

1. A primary object of linguistic research is to describe the precise minimal set of features sufficient to characterize all language sounds in a way that will bring out phonological patterns optimally; such a minimal set is called a set of *distinctive features.* In this chapter we are not concerned with whether a convenient descriptive feature is distinctive.

Variability in Production: Phonetic Detail

Laboratory measurements show that instances of "the same sound," like repetitions of any other natural event, are not completely identical. Instead, there is a range of tolerance for instances of, say, [d], which will all be taken as that sound despite variations in just where the front of the tongue touches the alveolar ridge, how long this closure lasts, and when the associated vocal cord vibration starts and stops. Outside this range of tolerance lie sounds that may be taken for a /d/ pronounced with some kind of foreign accent. The tongue tip may have been used instead of the slightly broader area that lies just behind it, the upper contact point may have been the back of the teeth or the roof of the mouth instead of the alveolar ridge, or the timing of the contact may be outside the English range.

The range of acceptability is affected by many factors. Among them are the nearby sounds in the word and a sound's position at the beginning, middle, or end of a word. For example, measurements show that a voiced stop or fricative in the middle of an English word generally has vocal cord vibration extending throughout the whole period of oral closure. However, the voicing for an initial voiced stop need not begin until about a fiftieth of a second after the closure has actually been released, and the voicing for a final voiced stop or fricative may die away well before the end of the oral closure. Some of these fine details are audible to the trained ear, but many of them are not, and instrumental analysis is required to study them.

Contrast: The Phoneme

On what grounds do we say that two audibly different sounds are both kinds of [t] but that another sound, objectively similar to them, is a [d] or a [k]? Native speakers of a language find such a question odd; we are normally quite sure that certain sounds are the same and others are different. Temporary confusion, however, may arise because of spelling, as in the two sounds [θ] and [ð], both spelled *th*. What we do to clear up that confusion is instructive. To show that there are two different sounds involved, we note that there are pairs of words, such as *thigh* and *thy*, that are kept distinct merely by the difference in pronunciation of the sounds in question. Such a pair of words, differing only with respect to one pair of sounds, is called a **minimal pair,** and two sounds are said to *contrast* if there is a minimal pair containing them.

A linguist studying an unknown language looks for minimal pairs to try to establish whether two similar sounds should be treated as variants of the same speech sound or as separate sounds. All the contrasting sounds in a language constitute its set of **phonemes.** The unvoiced [θ] and the voiced [ð] are separate phonemes in English, but there are other pairs of sounds differing in exactly the same way that are not in contrast and therefore do not represent separate phonemes. For example, the sound spelled *r* in *truck* or *cream*—more generally, *r* after any syllable-initial unvoiced stop— can be shown by instrumental analysis to be completely or largely unvoiced, although this is extremely difficult to hear. The voiced and unvoiced *r* do not contrast—there is no pair of words that is kept distinct by virtue of the fact that one contains a voiced *r* and the other contains its unvoiced variant, written with the symbol r̥. We speak of the two variants of *r* as being different **phones** but as representing the same phoneme, which we denote as /r/, using slanted lines. Square brackets are used to refer to phones; thus, the variants [r] and [r̥] are phones that represent the phoneme /r/. (Square brackets are also used to enclose the productions of young children.)

The distinction between phone and phoneme can be difficult to grasp, but the basic idea that some units of behavior are two concrete manifestations of the same abstract, socially defined unit can be found throughout anthropology. A dollar coin and a dollar bill are equivalent representations of a dollar value but contrast in value with coins and bills of other denominations; the queen on a chessboard plays the same role whether it is stamped of plastic or carved of ivory.

If any of several phones may be used to represent the same phoneme in a particular context, those phones are said to be in **free variation.** For example, in English, initial voiced stops may really have vocal cord vibration extending through their period of closure, but the voicing may also begin anywhere within about a fiftieth of a second after closure is relaxed. It makes no difference to the English listener whether the first (through-voiced) or the second (short-lag) phone is used. However, most linguistic variation is not free; some is stylistic and some is controlled by the linguistic context. We can go back to the "dollar" analogy: A vending machine will require coins, and a foreign currency exchange booth will accept only bills. Similarly, the unvoiced version of /r/ may be used only after unvoiced stops, and in fact it must be used there—English speakers typically have no control over the choice. In general, speakers find it very difficult to learn to hear the difference between two (or more) phones that belong to the same phoneme or to learn to override the automatic choice of which one to use in a given context. However, choice between separate phonemes is in general under voluntary control; one can choose to say "red" or to say "led." This is one of the reasons that the phoneme is taken as a basic behavioral unit of language and that many central questions in developmental phonology have been raised in terms of the phoneme.

Phonotactics: Possible and Impossible Words

So far we have talked about properties, such as voicing and the place of articulation, which are intrinsic characteristics of how each speech sound is made. Now we will consider the various sequences of English sounds that can be found and the positions of these sequences at the beginning, middle, or end of a word. This topic is called **phonotactics.**

Not every sequence of English sounds is a possible English word. No English word begins with the sound /ŋ/, which is why a set like *ram, ran, rang* had to be used to present the nasals in Table 3.1. If a new product were to be called Ngicekreem, it might be pronounced /nəgajskrim/ or /ɛŋgajskrim/, but only a few English speakers would be able to master the pronunciation /ŋajskrim/. We have the same problem with African names like Nkomo /ŋkomo/; this name is usually turned into /n-komo/ or /ɛnkomo/. And while English words frequently end with consonant clusters such as *lp* or *rt,* no English word can begin with either of these sound sequences. We can say *plot* and *true,* but we cannot have a word like *lpot* or *rtue.* Similarly, English words can begin with *pl* or *tr* but cannot end with those sequences, unless the *l* or *r* is used as a vowel as in *example* /ɛg-zæm-pl/. In French, however, words can end in such consonant clusters; the word *exemple* is pronounced /ɛk-sãmpl/ with the *l* an unvoiced consonant.

Phoneme sequence and position restrictions such as these are by no means random, although they do not seem to be completely regular. Therefore, instead of just listing permissible and impermissible sequences, we can make general statements with some notes of exception. The major initial consonant cluster restriction in English is that a word cannot begin with two stop consonants in a row, but most initial sequences of a stop followed by a liquid, /s/ followed by a stop, and /s/ plus stop plus liquid are pronounceable, as in *true, stew,* and *strew* respectively.

In learning a second language, mastering a new cluster or a new word position for a familiar sound may require quite as much work as mastering an entirely new sound. English speakers learning Russian usually have problems with monosyllabic words like *rta* (mouth) and *lba* (forehead) as well as *vzglyad* (glance). It turns out, similarly, that learning new phonotactic arrangements is as central a part of the child's acquisition of phonology as is the learning of individual phonemes.

Morphophonology

Morphemes

To understand morphophonology, we must also consider the important concepts of **morpheme** and **allomorph.** Words often can be seen to consist of smaller meaningful parts; the smallest units that carry meaning are called *morphemes.* Any word that cannot be subdivided into smaller parts with meaning is therefore a morpheme: *hat, run, big, how. Hatband, runner, biggest,* and *however* consist of two morphemes each. The *-er* of *runner* and the *-est* of *biggest* are separable, meaningful elements; *-er* here means "one who," and *-est* means "most." The inflectional endings, like the *-s* that signals plural and the *-d* that indicates past tense, are also morphemes that cannot stand alone. English has a much smaller set of these endings than languages like Latin, German, or French.

Allomorphy in Inflectional Endings

Some inflectional endings have the same shape regardless of the words they are attached to, like the progressive *-ing* of verbs like *giving.* Others, however, have different shapes depending on the sound of the word or stem that they are attached to.

These different shapes are called the *allomorphs* of the morpheme, and *morphophonology* describes the way that the choice among allomorphs is determined. The plural morpheme, for example, sounds like /s/ when it follows unvoiced stops: *cats, rocks.* When the plural morpheme follows a vowel or voiced stops, its sound is /z/: *days, kids, dogs.* There is one group of final sounds that requires still a third variant of this morpheme. Words ending in the hissing or sibilant sounds /s/, /z/, /ʃ/, /ʒ/, /tʃ/, or /dʒ/ take the variant [əz]—*kisses, sneezes, fishes, garages, churches,* and *judges.* These three variants of the plural morpheme are referred to as its *regular allomorphs;* regular, in this case, means that if one knows the sound of the singular noun, the choice among the three plural endings is automatic. There are also some irregular plural allomorphs, which have to be separately learned: for example, the *-en* of *oxen,* the *-ren* of *children,* and the internal vowel changes that signal the plural of words like *man.* (*Men,* therefore, consists of two morphemes, *man* and the plural, even though it can't be separated into stem and ending as *cats* can.) There are also some words like *sheep* and *deer* that are unchanged in the plural; such words are said to have a zero plural allomorph when they are used with plural meaning.

Allomorphy in Other Morphemes

English has other morphemes that are found almost entirely in words inherited or derived from Greek and Latin origins. Some of these also exhibit allomorphy; that is, the same morpheme will have several allomorphs. For example, the adjective ending - *ic* (*electric, toxic*) is found in the form /ɪk/ when it stands at the end of a word or before certain other endings, but in the allomorph /ɪs/ when the noun-forming *-ity* is added to it, as in *electricity* or *toxicity.*

The form variations that we have discussed so far have all involved forms of word endings. The inflections (plural, past) showed different allomorphs depending on what base word (stem) they were attached to, and the adjective ending *-ic* showed up as /ɪs/ when the additional noun-forming ending *-ity* was attached to it. The stem of a word may also vary when an ending is attached. Consider the pronunciation (not the spelling) of the following verb–noun pairs, which show **stem allomorphy.**

Verb	Noun	Verb	Noun
inflate	inflation	abrade	abrasion
relate	relation	invade	invasion
pollute	pollution	delude	delusion
promote	promotion	corrode	corrosion

There seems to be an ending spelled *-ion* that turns these verbs into nouns, but the final consonant in the verb also changes in pronunciation when *-ion* is added. The morphemes ending in /t/, such as *promote,* show alternate forms with /ʃ/ in the related nouns; the morphemes ending in /d/, like *corrode,* show alternates ending in /ʒ/. We might try to link what happens to /t/ and what happens to /d/ by saying that alveolar consonants before *-ion* become palatal fricatives but do not change their voicing.

As we explore the English lexicon, however, we run into problems with formulating an explicit rule connecting a verb with its allomorph in an *-ion* noun. *Insert* gives *insertion,* with /ʃ/, but *invert* gives *inversion,* with /ʒ/; *degrade* gives *degradation,* not *degrasion; collect* gives *collection,* but *suspect* gives *suspicion,* not *suspection.* Many verbs have no *-ion* form at all (although one could imagine what such a related noun ought to be like): there is no *debation* or *debasion* to correspond to *debate.* Finally, there are many *-ion* nouns with no corresponding English verb: there is *vision* but not *vide, occasion* but not *occade.*

Recognition of Allomorphic Relations

In English, stem allomorphy involves many more irregularities and gaps than affix allomorphy. The question is often raised (Braine, 1974) as to whether English speakers apprehend these relationships at all since they have to memorize the proper noun and verb forms anyway. Furthermore, if speakers do sense correspondence between such pairs of words, can they be said to know rules expressing that correspondence in anything like the way they know rules linking the regular /s/, /z/, and /əz/ allomorphs of the plural?

Research (Jaeger, 1980; Myerson, 1975; Wilbur & Menn, 1975) indicates that speakers may indeed apprehend many of the less regular relationships between allomorphs, especially with the help of hints embodied in English spelling (the orthographic resemblance between *ignite* and *ignition* may facilitate recognition of their relationship). However, speakers do not have to extract the intricate patterns that we have just surveyed in order to become competent users of English since one does not have to make up new *-ion* words and, in fact, must refrain from doing so: spiting someone is not *spition,* nor is avoiding *avoision.* We say, therefore, that *-ion* is not a **productive** ending in English. In contrast, the regular plural, past, progressive, and possessive endings are productive. They can be added to almost any word, and especially to new words, if the semantics of the occasion demand.

Stress and Intonation Contour

The **stress** or accent pattern within a word is intimately related to the sounds in it, especially to the vowel sounds. In English, vowels are longer, louder, and often higher in pitch when they are in stressed (accented) syllables than when they are in unstressed syllables. In addition, if adding an ending to a word causes the stress to shift from one syllable to another, some of the vowels in the word may change more drastically and actually become different phonemes. These changes are often not reflected in spelling. For example, when the word *declare* /də-klejr/ is used to make *declaration* /dɛ-klə-réj-ʃn/, the stress changes: /kléjr/ loses its stress, /də/ gains a little, and the strongest accent goes to the third syllable. Other examples of stress shifting when an ending is added can be seen in pairs like *méthod–methódical* and *nórmal–normálity*; in each case the vowels are affected. Endings may also trigger changes in vowels even when the stress does not shift; consider pairs like *vain–vánity* or *south–southern.*

In constructing sentences, stress has many uses that are beyond the scope of this chapter; the most familiar is probably contrastive or emphatic stress, as when one says, "I want the bláck book, not the green book," with the strongest stresses on *black* and *green.* Compare this sentence with "I want the black book, not the black notebook"; in the latter the strongest stresses are on the first *book* and on *note.* Another use of stress in English is to distinguish compounds from phrases: *greénhouse* (transparent structure for growing plants) is a compound and is stressed on the word *green,* but a *green house* is any house painted green, and when there is no occasion for emphasis on the color, the word *house* bears greater or at least equal stress—"At the end of this road there's a green house and then a pond."

In this particular pair spelling distinguishes the compound *greenhouse* from the phrase *green house;* however, orthography is not reliable since, for example, the compound *hót dog* (frankfurter) is spelled the same as the phrase *hot dóg* (a very warm canine pet). There are also some items, like *apple pie* and *chocolate cake,* that can be thought of either as compounds or as phrases; some speakers stress these on the first word and some on the second.

The pitch or melody of the voice rises and falls during speaking, and the pattern of pitch changes accompanying a phrase or sentence is called its **intonation contour.** Strong final rises in pitch are found in many (but not all!) types of questions, and smaller rises are often found in tentative polite statements. A rise in pitch corresponds to an increase in frequency of vocal cord vibration, and this can easily be measured in the laboratory.

Conversational Speech and Regional Variants

In conversational speech, the pronunciation of words may differ very strongly from the way the same words are produced when they are read aloud carefully from a list, but speakers are generally quite unaware of this fact. For example, in the phrase "I have to leave now," the *have* and *to* are always run together as a single word, pronounced [hæftə]; *want to* and *going to* are rendered as *wanna* or *wannu* and *gonna* or *gonnu,* except when they are being specially emphasized. In the conversational insert phrase *y'know,* many speakers reduce the sounds to something like [jõ]; the word *no* has a huge set of variants, which we sometimes try to write in English orthography as *naw, nah,* and the like.

Other common casual speech rules or processes in English include simplification of various word-final consonant clusters depending on how the next word begins ("George an' Mary"; "cann' peaches"), omission of vowels in unstressed syllables, partial devoicing of phrase-final voiced stops and fricatives, omission of /ð/ and /h/ in unstressed object pronouns ("I see 'er"; "Push 'em over here"), and so on.

Regional and Stylistic Variants

Most of us have lived only in a few areas of our native countries, and so we tend to have a very limited idea of the variations of English spoken in other regions, let alone in other English-speaking countries. Advertisement and entertainment media may give us a superficial acquaintance with stereotypes of the American southern, New York, Australian, or Cockney varieties of English, but such stereotypes represent only a few of the most striking differences between these varieties of English and what may be called the broadcasting network standard of the U.S. A few rough regional characteristics are listed below, but the best way to learn how people of a region really speak is to go there, tape, and listen to the fine details of their speech production.

A Few Regional Characteristics of American English. In the Midwest and West, the vowels [a] and [ɔ] contrast before [r]—*car* and *core* are distinct—but before sounds other than [r], these vowels are both produced as [a]: *cot* and *caught* are both [kat].

In the Middle Atlantic states, *cot* has the vowel [a] and *caught* has pretty much the same vowel [ɔ] as *core.*

In much of the Northeast, the vowels of *Mary, merry,* and *marry* are differentiated from one another as [meri], [mɛri], and [mæri], but in most of the rest of the country, two or all three of these words are homonyms, that is, are pronounced exactly the same way.

In much of the central part of the U.S., the vowels [ɪ] and [ɛ] are not distinguished before nasal consonants; *pin* and *pen,* for example, are homonyms, so that one may be asked, "Do you mean a [pɪən] to write with or a [pɪən] to fasten something with?"

In New York and New England, as well as much of the South, [r] is not pronounced at the ends of phrases nor before consonants. The [r] is often replaced by a lengthening, off-glide, or change of quality on the vowel preceding the position that it would have appeared in—for example, in some Boston-area speakers, the pronunciation of *shark* is [ʃa:k]. The vowel written [a:] is a long low front vowel, lower than the [æ] of *shack* [ʃæk] and farther front than the [a] of *shock* [ʃak].

In the New York area, a [g] is pronounced where it is written after [ŋ], but in the rest of the U.S., there is no [g] after [ŋ] at the ends of words, nor in nouns (e.g., *singer*) derived from verbs ending in [ŋ].

In the East, many words written with *or* (e.g., *orange, horrible*) are pronounced with [ar] rather than [ɔr]; however this is not true for all such words—*orchid* has [ɔr], for example.

In most of the U.S., [e], [i], [o], and [u] are **diphthongized,** that is, produced with a following off-glide as approximately [ej, ij, ow, uw], while [ɪ], [ɛ], and [ʊ] are **monophthongs;** however, in much of the South and Texas, the vowels in the first group are generally less diphthongized, while the vowels in the second set all tend to have a [ə] off-glide: *pan* is roughly [pæən].

In and near the large northern cities, the low vowels [æ] and [ɔ] are becoming more and more diphthongized, and the first part of the diphthong is becoming higher than it is in the rest of the U.S., so that they are approximately [eə] (or even [iə]) and [uə]. The names *Ann* and *Ian* are homophonous for many speakers in this region.

Stylistic Variation. A given person's pronunciation of a word also depends on the speech style being used at a given time. There is usually considerable variation between the highly self-monitored speech styles used for reading word fists aloud and presenting a new word to a young child, on the one hand, and the very unmonitored style used in a deeply involving conversation among family members or old friends, on the other hand. It is in the less monitored style that the most distinctive regional variations are most likely to be heard. Study of the details of such variations is one focus of the field of **sociolinguistics.**

Infant Speech Perception

To determine what infants perceive, researchers first needed to figure out a way of measuring babies' perceptual abilities. A number of ingenious techniques have been devised based on observations of the infant's physiological or behavioral responses to various sorts of auditory stimuli. One of the most successful techniques for studying the abilities of infants in the first few months after birth is **high amplitude sucking** (HAS). In this method, the infant is given a pacifier to suck on that is connected to a sound generating system. Each suck causes a noise to be generated and the infant learns quickly that sucking brings about this noise. At first, babies suck frequently and the noise occurs often; then, gradually, they lose interest in hearing repetitions of the same noise and begin to suck less frequently. At this point, the experimenter changes the sound that is being generated. If the babies renew vigorous sucking, it can be inferred that they have discriminated the sound change and are sucking more in response to their interest in a new and different sound.

With this technique, researchers have been able to gain information about perceptual abilities of very young infants. We now know that even in the first few months, infants can discriminate many fine distinctions between speech sounds. For example, Eimas and colleagues (Eimas, Siqueland, Jusczyk, & Vigorito, 1971) demonstrated that infants as young as one month of age are capable of perceiving the distinction between /b/ and /p/ in the syllables /ba/ and /pa/, although the difference in these sounds is minimal: /b/ differs from /p/ only in that vocal cord vibration starts sometime less than about one twenty-fifth of a second after the lips are opened for /b/, but sometime more than after one twenty-fifth of a second after the lips are opened for /p/. Interestingly, the infants' discrimination of these sounds was **categorical,** as it is in adults; that is, the infants discriminated the difference in vocal cord vibration delay (**voice onset time**) between /b/ and /p/, but ignored similar-sized timing differences involving different tokens within the categories of /b/ or /p/ (e.g., they did not start sucking more frequently when the sound changed from /ba/ with a through-voiced [b] to /ba/ with a short-lag [b]).

It has also been shown that infants under three months can detect differences in place and manner of articulation of consonants, and in contrasting intonational patterns [see Jusczyk (1992) for a summary of these studies]. The fact that infants can discriminate between very similar speech sounds at one month of age would suggest either that they have a built-in ability to make such distinctions or that they learn them very quickly. One way to test between these two alternative explanations is to look at a sound discrimination that infants could never have learned—that is, one that is not used in the language to which they have been exposed. Trehub (1976) ran such a study, testing Canadian infants who had not been exposed to any eastern European language for their discrimination of two fairly similar sounds used in Czech, [ʒa] and [řa]. Adult Canadian subjects were also tested for their ability to differentiate the two unfamiliar sounds. Although infants could discriminate [ʒa] and [řa] as well as they could English language contrasts such as [ba] and [pa], the English-speaking adults readily confused the Czech sounds.

The results of Trehub's study suggest not only that infants are born with the ability to hear the difference between the Czech phonemes, but that language experience may result in the loss of the ability to discriminate categories that are not functional in one's language. This possibility is supported by the results of another study of English-learning infants. Werker and Tees (1984) found that between six and eight months the infants could discriminate sounds that are used in Hindi or Nthlakapmx (a Salish language spoken in Canada) but not in English. By ten to twelve months, this discrimination ability had disappeared, and the infants' performance was as poor as that of English-speaking adults.

In a series of cross-linguistic studies on the perception of vowels, Kuhl (1992) has demonstrated that infants reared in different linguistic environments show an effect of language experience by six months of age. Specifically, infants begin to group vowels differently, reflecting language-specific characteristics of the ambient language input.

It appears, then, that infants start out the language-acquisition process with the capacity to discriminate the phonetic contrasts of any of the world's languages. With exposure to their own language, they begin to focus on those contrasts that are relevant for that particular language, and to lose the ability to perceive certain contrasts not found in their native language. However, this does not mean that infants (or adults) fail to distinguish among all nonnative contrasts; for instance, both English-learning babies of fourteen months and English-speaking adults can perceive differences among clicks in Zulu, even though these sounds do not occur in English (Best, McRoberts, & Sithole, 1988). It seems that the decline in discrimination abilities affects primarily those foreign sounds that are phonetically similar, though not identical, to sounds of the native language.

Some of the most intriguing findings in the field of infant speech perception involve studies of infants' abilities in the first week of life. DeCasper and Fifer (1980), for example, showed that three-day-old infants can identify their own mothers' voices when presented with voices of various mothers; moreover, there was evidence that they prefer listening to their own mother than to another mother. Mehler and his colleagues (Mehler et al., 1988) demonstrated that four-day-old infants can distinguish between utterances in their maternal language and those of another language. In both cases, it appears likely that the discrimination abilities are based primarily on prosodic cues in the utterances (such cues could be perceived in the uterus) rather than phonetic features of particular sounds.

Production: The Prelinguistic Period

During the first year of life, infants produce a variety of vocalizations, beginning with simple cries at birth and progressing through an ordered sequence of stages to complex babbling with identifiable syllables and adultlike intonation patterns. The productions can be divided into two general categories: (1) **reflexive** vocalizations—cries, coughs, and involuntary grunts that seem to be automatic responses reflecting the physical state of the infant—and (2) **nonreflexive** vocalizations, like *cooing* or *jargon babbling*—nonautomatic productions containing many phonetic features found in adult languages.

Regardless of the linguistic community in which they are being raised, all infants seem to pass through the same stages of vocal development. In this section, we will describe these stages and the approximate ages associated with each, using the frameworks of Oller (1980) and Stark (1980). (These are slightly more elaborate than the list presented in Chapter 2.) Although commonly referred to as "stages," the periods described here are not discrete; that is, vocalization types typically overlap from one stage to another. A new stage is marked by the appearance of vocal behaviors not observed in the preceding period.

Stage 1.

Reflexive vocalizations (birth to two months). This stage is characterized by a majority of reflexive vocalizations, such as crying and fussing, and vegetative sounds like coughing, burping, and sneezing. In addition, some vowel-like sounds may occur. The vocalizations of this period are partially determined by the infant's anatomical structure. In newborn babies, the vocal tract resembles that of a nonhuman primate in that the oral cavity is small and almost totally filled by the tongue, and the larynx is high in the neck, with little separation of the oral and nasal cavities (Lieberman, Crelin, & Klatt, 1972). This configuration limits the range of sound types that can be produced. Rapid growth of the head and neck area in the stages that follow allows production of a greater variety of sounds.

Stage 2.

Cooing and laughter (two to four months). During this stage, infants begin to make some comfort-state vocalizations, often called *cooing* or *gooing* sounds. As indicated by this label, these vocalizations seem to be made in the back of the mouth, with velar consonants and back vowels. Crying typically becomes less frequent and, much to parents' delight, sustained laughter and infant chuckles appear.

Stage 3.

Vocal play (four to six months). In this period it seems as though babies are testing their vocal apparatus to determine the range of vocal qualities they can produce. The period is characterized by the appearance of very loud and very soft sounds (yells and whispers), and very high and very low sounds (squeals and growls). Some babies produce long series of raspberries (bilabial trills) and sustained vowels, and occasionally some rudimentary syllables of consonants and vowels occur.

Stage 4.

Canonical babbling (six months and older). The prime feature of this period is the appearance of sequences of consonant–vowel syllables with adultlike timing. For the first time, babies sound as though they are actually trying to produce words. Upon hearing a sequence such as [mama] or [dada], parents often report with delight that their baby has begun to call them by name. To be sure, it does sound as though the baby is saying *mama* or *daddy;* in most cases, however, there is no evidence that the productions are semantically linked to an identifiable referent, so for this reason these forms would not be considered words. Multisyllabic utterances in this period are often categorized as **reduplicated babbles** (i.e., strings of identical syllables like [bababa]) or **variegated babbles** (syllable strings with varying consonants and vowels, like [bagidabu]). While both types of utterances occur in the canonical stage, reduplicated babbles predominate initially; around twelve or thirteen months, variegated babbles emerge as the more frequent type.

The infant's hearing of his own vocalizations and the vocalizations of those around him takes on increased importance during this period. We know this because although deaf infants engage in the earlier forms of vocalization, they fail to enter the canonical babbling stage at the appropriate time (Oller & Eilers, 1988). Moreover, during this period the variety of consonants in the vocalizations of deaf infants decreases with age, whereas the variety increases with age in the vocalizations of hearing babies (Stoel-Gammon & Otomo, 1986).

Stage 5.

Jargon stage (ten months and older). The last stage of babbling overlaps with the early period of meaningful speech, and is characterized by strings of sounds and syllables uttered with a rich variety of stress and intonational patterns. This kind of output is known by such names as *conversational babble, modulated babble,* or *jargon.* To many adults it seems as though children are speaking in whole sentences—making statements, asking questions—but are using their "own" language rather than the standard language spoken by the older children and adults around them.

This impression comes from more than the sounds themselves; it also comes from other aspects of the children's behavior. Many vocalizations are delivered with eye contact, gesture, and intonation so rich and appropriate that the person addressed typically feels compelled to respond, at least with a neutral "You don't say" or "How nice." More objectively, a child producing conversational babble seems to have a full grasp of the social nature of conversation and has merely missed the fact that the sounds in it have particular meanings. It is not generally correct, however, to call such conversational babble meaningless, because the gestures and the context often make it clear that the intonation—the rise and fall of the pitch of the voice—is indeed carrying meaning even if the articulated sounds are not. Thus, the term **modulated babble** is also used to refer to these conversational vocalizations. Conversational babble can clearly convey requests for aid, rejection of food or toys, or desire to direct attention to ongoing events (Menn, 1976). On the other hand, sometimes the child is apparently not conveying any meaning by her eloquent use of intonation contour; sometimes she appears to be simply imitating the outward form of adult conversation as an end in itself, for example, in pretended telephone conversations.

Some vocalizations appear to be made for their own sake. The child does not appear to be "talking" to anyone, and there seems to be no connection between the sounds and any other ongoing activity. Such **sound play** may contain recurring favorite sound sequences, or even early words.

Sounds of Babbling

The speechlike sounds used by infants change dramatically during the first year of life. In the first six months, vowel articulations tend to predominate; as mentioned above, most consonantal sounds are produced in the back of the mouth (i.e., sounds like [k] or [g]). With the onset of the canonical babbling stage, there is a marked shift toward front consonants, particularly [m], [b], and [d].

Between six and twelve months, the sound repertoire expands considerably. However, claims that babies produce all the sounds of all languages of the world (Jakobson, 1941/1968) in this period have not been substantiated. In fact, studies have shown that a relatively small set of consonants accounts for the great majority of consonantal sounds produced. In his review of babbling data from 129 infants aged eleven to twelve months, Locke (1983) showed that twelve of the twenty-four consonantal sounds of English accounted for nearly 95 percent of the consonants produced. In terms of articulatory features, this set of sounds is characterized by particular manner classes, namely the stops [p, b, t, d, k, g], the nasals [m, n], and the glides [w, j]; in addition, the fricative [s] and the glottal [h] are included in the list. Interestingly, the sound classes that are missing from babble—fricatives like [v] or [ð], affricates like [tʃ], and liquids [l] and [r]—are precisely those classes of sounds that are mastered relatively late in the production of *real words;* in contrast, the consonants that are frequent in late babbling (the stops, nasals, and glides) are nearly identical to those that appear in the first adult-based words (Stoel-Gammon, 1985). Thus, it seems that the sounds of late babbling may serve as the building blocks for the production of words. Although there is a fair amount of individual variation, on average, stops, nasals, and glides appear in children's words before fricatives, affricates, and liquids.

The Relationship between Babbling and Speech

At one time, it was suggested that early attempts at speech grew directly out of bab- bling, in response to adult language teaching. The idea was that infants babbled all possible sounds and that adults selectively reinforced those sounds that occurred in the input language and ignored sounds that did not (Mowrer, 1954; Winitz, 1969). There are several problems with this view. First, babies do not start out producing all possible sounds; they produce only a relatively small subset of them (Oller, 1980). Second, even though studies have shown that adult attention can increase the amount of babbling, it does not change the type of sounds that are produced (Dodd, 1972; Rheingold, Gerwitz, & Ross, 1959; Todd & Palmer, 1968; Wahler, 1969; Weisberg, 1963). Finally, babbled sounds do not markedly change to become more like the input language. A number of studies have examined whether listeners or spectro- graphic analyses could distinguish the babbled sounds of babies who have been exposed to different languages, and the results have consistently shown that the sounds are very similar, even with input languages as different as English, Arabic, Spanish, Japanese, and Chinese (Atkinson, MacWhinney, & Stoel, 1970; Nakazima, 1962; Olney & Scholnick, 1976). Only when judges listened to longer segments of babbling that contained intonational cues could they recognize babies from their own speech communities (Boysson-Bardies, Sagart, & Durand, 1984).

Another theory about the relationship between babbling and speech was that the two stages were essentially discontinuous. Jesperson (1925) proposed that bab- bling consisted of the playful exploration of the sounds that the baby could make, whereas speech involved the "planful" execution of particular sounds. Jakobson (1941/1968) developed this idea, suggesting that in babbling the infant randomly produced a wide range of sounds but could use only a restricted set of sounds when speech began. Furthermore, he had observed that some children had a "silent period" when babbling ceased just before true speech began.

More recently, evidence has suggested that the best way to characterize the rela- tionship between babbling and speech is the *continuity* view. Detailed longitudinal studies of prelinguistic vocalizations have shown that children's phonological patterns in early meaningful speech are directly linked to the patterns they used in babbling. Although there are universal trends in terms of sound classes, as we noted above, the presence of individual preferences in babbling has also been documented, and these same preferences appear in the child's first words (Vihman, Macken, Miller, Sim- mons, & Miller, 1985; Vihman, 1996). Early words tend to use the same sounds that the child has preferred in babbling, presumably because these are the sounds that she has managed to bring under voluntary control. Early speech develops gradually out of babbling, and typically coexists with it for several months at least.

Another factor in support of the continuity view is the recent evidence showing an influence of the ambient language on babbling patterns. Studies of children acquiring French, English, Swedish, or Japanese have shown that they tend to use the same types of sounds, but that there are systematic differences in the frequency of occurrence of particular sound classes (Boysson-Bardies & Vihman, 1991). These differences in proportional occurrence mirror the proportional use of sounds in the children's early words, showing evidence, once again, of a continuity between the sound patterns of babbling and those of early speech.

The Beginning of Phonological Development: Protowords

The beginning of speech seems easy to identify for some children. One day they make a sound that resembles an adult word, and they do it when that word would be appropriate. These first recognizable words are often greetings, farewells, or other social phrases, like "peek-a-boo." The situation is more problematic when the child has a recurrent form that doesn't resemble any appropriate adult word; for example, Halliday's (1975) subject Nigel created several of his own forms, such as the "na" used to indicate that he wanted an object. Does a word that the child has made up "count?"

It does, in at least two respects. First, the child who uses such a form has demonstrated an important level of voluntary control over his vocalizations, a level that is necessary (though perhaps not sufficient) for starting to say words that do have adult models. Second, a child using one or two invented words has acquired the difficult concept that sounds have meaning and is unclear only about the fact that you are supposed to find out what words exist instead of making them up for yourself.

The term **protoword** is often used for the invented words that may occur during the transition from prespeech to speech; it is also sometimes used for carry words that have adult models but lack important semantic properties of those models. However, consideration of that topic will take us too far away from the acquisition of phonology. [The Halliday (1975) and Painter (1984) case studies are recommended for those who wish to explore this area further.]

Protowords (with or without adult models) often differ in another way from our usual notion of a word; although the sound sequences must be stable enough so that one can identify their recurrences (otherwise an adult would never realize that a child intended the sounds to have a particular meaning), they may be very poorly controlled, and individual instances may vary much more than repeated uses of a word do in adult usage. For example, Menn's (1976) subject Jacob had an identifiable proto-word that he used to accompany the action of rotating anything that would turn (a wheel, a knob, a page of a book); the form of this "spinning song" varied from "ioioio" to "weeaweeaweea."

Theories of the Acquisition of Phonology

Until about 1970, two kinds of theories of phonological development existed in sharp conflict, one **nativist** and the other **behaviorist**. A nativist theory of development holds that normal development proceeds like the development of an embryo; the environment provides raw materials that are assimilated and structured by the child according to an inborn program. The opposite theoretical pole is a behaviorist theory, which holds that the biological heritage is only anatomical—it determines, for example, the shape of the vocal tract, the auditory processing mechanism, and other physical characteristics that support language. All language behavior is held to be learned by stimulus-reward experience; children's word approximations are shaped by the reward of getting what they ask for until their forms match adult models.

Nativist Theory

The best-known nativist theory was put forward by the late Roman Jakobson (1941/1968). Jakobson's theory was based on theoretical considerations drawn from adult language and from the few then-available reports of children's early words, and it is now known to be inadequate in several important respects. However, his work was of great importance because of the interest it aroused in child phonology, especially his claim that sounds that are acquired late in any given language are those that are relatively rare in the languages of the world.

Jakobson's theory was really rather limited in scope; it dealt only with the order of phonemic contrasts developed by children, and it does, indeed, appear to describe this in broad outline. His notion was that all children should show essentially the same order of acquisition of phonemic contrasts and that the earliest contrasts developed by the individual should be those that are most common in the languages of the world. Therefore, children would first learn to produce the consonant–vowel contrast since that is found in all languages—syllables like "pa-pa" and "ma-ma," which of course many children do say. He proposed that children would then proceed to subdivide both vowels and consonants, making finer and finer distinctions until they reached the full set of contrasts demanded by the language around them. The subdivision of consonants was supposed to begin either by distinguishing nasal from nonnasal stops or labial from nonlabial stops; after the labial–nonlabial contrast had been acquired, a child could learn to distinguish back (usually velar) consonants from dental or alveolar ones.

While this order of development is fairly common, counterexamples have been published. Menn (1976) followed a child named Jacob from age twelve to twenty-one months and showed that he acquired a contrast between dental and velar stops before learning to produce labials. Other children who have been studied—for example, Hildegard (Leopold, 1970)—have produced a word without any vowel, like "mmm" or "shhh," as a first word. This contradicts the mama-papa prediction. We note again that Jakobson's theory says nothing about phones in themselves but only as they represent phonemes, so the development of phonetic accuracy simply falls outside the scope of his theory.

Behaviorist Theory

The behaviorist approach to the acquisition of phonology is best exemplified by the work of Olmsted (1971). Olmsted was concerned with phones, not phonemic contrasts, and he tried to show that children tended to begin acquisition with the most frequent phones of their language and then proceed to the least frequent ones. It seems to have been assumed that the reward for improved approximation of each phone should be roughly equal. This theory, like Jakobson's, doesn't account for the degree of individual variation that children show in the order of acquisition of phones; in addition, it is contradicted by the fact that the very frequent phone [ð] is among the last to be acquired. Clearly, some phones, like [ð], are harder to learn to say than others, either for perceptual or articulatory reasons.

More importantly, there is a counterargument that works against both nativist and behaviorist types of theories, at least in the forms in which they have been advocated. Both nativist and behaviorist theories predict that development will follow a course of smooth, regular improvement toward an adult model, without any regression. But we know of clear cases of regression in the acquisition of phonology.

Regression: Key Evidence against Both Nativist and Behaviorist Theories

Menn's (1971) study of the acquisition of phonology provides an example of a child who clearly showed **regression;** the pronunciation of two frequently used words actually got worse over time. Daniel established the words *down* and *stone* as [dæwn] (correct) and [don] ("doan"). Then, however, when he tried to say other words beginning with oral stops and ending in nasals, he produced them with nasals in both positions. For example, he produced beans as [minz] ("means") and dance as [næns] ("nance"). After a few weeks this nasal assimilation began to take over the established forms for *down* and *stone;* soon he was saying [næwn] ("noun") and [non] ("noan"). Behaviorist theories must assume that correct forms are rewarded more than incorrect ones; therefore, they cannot deal with the replacement of correct forms with incorrect ones.

Another type of regression doesn't involve a particular word getting worse, but rather the apparent loss of the ability to say a sound in new words, coupled with retention of the correct pronunciation in older words. This variability is also in itself evidence against a strong nativist theory. For example, many children acquire a word or two whose pronunciation is much closer to the adult model than that of their other words. These words were called **progressive phonological idioms** by Moskowitz (1980). Menn's Daniel had initial [h] only on his second and third words, *hi* and *hello;* all other adult words beginning with /h/, for example *horse, hose, hat*—indeed, all adult words beginning with glides, liquids, or fricatives—were produced without the initial semivowel or consonant. The ability to begin words with [h] appears to have been acquired and maintained for the two words *hi* and *hello* but to have been absent in all other cases. It would be impossible to speak of Daniel either as having learned to produce [h] or as not having done so. No strictly nativist model can be flexible enough to deal with this kind of word-to-word variation. There is no linguistic way to predict which words will become progressive phonological idioms and which words will not.

Cognitive Approaches to the Acquisition of Phonology

The sort of theory of phonological development that seems to deal best with the data reported here is called a *cognitive* or *problem-solving* theory, for in it the child is seen as a somewhat intelligent creature actively trying to solve a difficult problem: how to talk like the people around her do (Macken & Ferguson, 1983). She may adopt several general strategies that can provide temporary solutions: avoidance of difficult sounds or sound sequences, exploitation of favorite sounds, systematic replacement or less systematic rearrangement of the sounds in the target word. She may also have a general one-word-at-a-time approach or instead try to approximate whole phrases.

Within a child's general strategy, one can see characteristic components of problem solving: first, trial-and-error articulation attempts, but then the use of existing solutions to deal with new problems (generalization), and the temporary extension of these behaviors to situations where they are not quite the needed response (overgeneralization), like Daniel's use of "noun" for *down*. This sequence of events is typical of all areas of linguistic development and is a major reason for considering language development to be a part of general cognitive development.

Before leaving the discussion of the older theories, let us see what they do have of continuing value. Both contain elements that must be incorporated into any adequate approach. Nativist theories highlight the fact that the raw materials—the brain and the perceptual and motor systems, including their patterns of postnatal maturation—are biologically given. These put limits, some absolute and some probabilistic, on behavior, and many of the similarities among children are surely to be accounted for by this biological "substrate" for language. For example, the perceptual system will respond to the acoustic similarities between the fricatives /s/ and /ʃ/; a child learning to say them by trial and error may therefore be satisfied temporarily by the same sound for both of them. Another example: Stops in general seem easier to produce than fricatives—perhaps because a stop can be produced by a fairly clumsy lip or tongue gesture since what is needed is a complete closure of the oral passage. However, the production of a fricative needs more delicate motor control: Just the right distance to cause airstream turbulence must be maintained between the upper and lower articulators, and the right airstream speed as well. All this is a matter of physiology and physics.

Such considerations of innate predispositions and abilities are most often helpful when we look for explanations of what children tend to have in common. We need to modify the old absolute statements, however, giving them a probabilistic cast (e.g., "It is more likely that a child will use a stop for a fricative than vice versa" rather than "Stops are mastered before fricatives"). General statements about the order of acquisition of particular segments also have to be made in probabilistic terms; the order varies across children, and the actual ages of acquisition vary even more.

When we look for explanations of how children differ from each other, it is also not surprising to find that there is a useful role for behaviorist notions of trial-and-error shaped by reward. But again, the problem-solving theory gives the behaviorist idea an important new twist, for the notion of where rewards come from has changed. Traditional behaviorism assumes that the reward for correct behavior is external. The successful communication of a demand is rewarded when the child gets what he wants and thus learns to say the word(s) the same way the next time.

The real-life problems in this theory become glaringly obvious in any kitchen where a semi-intelligible child is trying to get a cookie; a child at this stage gets most of what she wants by whine, gaze, and gesture. This gives little occasion for differential reinforcement of any kind of articulatory improvement, and parental injunctions to "say *cookie*" are seldom heeded by the child who really wants one.

There is also a much stronger counterargument to the external-reward theory. If external reward were the principal shaper of behavior, prelingually deaf children would not have such a terribly difficult time learning to use spoken language. A deaf child in an oral training program is given intensive feedback from teachers, and yet many never learn to produce a useful amount of intelligible speech, although fully effective communication through manual sign language can be learned rapidly if the child has parents and companions who communicate with one of the sign languages used by the deaf community.

What is lacking in the deaf child's learning of speech but present in his acquisition of sign language? Clearly, because he cannot hear, he cannot monitor his own performance and match it against the models provided by others. The missing element, in other words, is *internal feedback*. Learning the intricate motor skill of speaking (like any other fine motor skill) requires the ability to assess one's own performance. Imagine learning to play tennis if you had to rely on someone else to tell you where the ball went! A deaf child can see his hands and the hands of others in order to judge the accuracy of his signs, but he cannot hear his words or compare them to the words of others and so cannot judge the accuracy of his sounds.

It is quite obvious why there is such a difference in effectiveness between internal and external feedback. There are literally dozens—even hundreds—of phonetic details that must fall within narrow tolerances for production of an adult-sounding word. The language learner must be able to tell, consciously or unconsciously, what part of a word is wrong and to play around with it, listening to it until she gets it better. So, the reward for a closer approximation of the adult form must be the child's own realization that she has "gotten" it; she must be pleased with herself for sounding more like her family or her friends. (For evidence that children practice their words and sounds, see Ferguson & Macken, 1980; Weir, 1962.)

The problem-solving theory, in summary, assumes that most of the reward is internal; the child is innately disposed to feel pleasure with behavior that he apprehends as successful emulation of adult or peer models. One current research endeavor is the attempt to construct computer models of the **self-organizing system** type, using internal feedback, to see if they can indeed simulate early phonological development (Leonard, 1992; Lindblom, 1992; Menn & Matthei, 1992; Stemberger 1992).

Learning to Pronounce

How do very young children really pronounce their words? Let us consider the examples from published literature found in Table 3.3. Some productions are quite accurate, others show overall resemblances between the target and the attempt, and some seem a little farfetched. But beyond displaying a list of examples, what more can be said? If there is some order behind this variety, how can it be elucidated?

Regularity in Children's Renditions of Adult Words

One of the most important findings from the study of the acquisition of phonology is that most of the young children who have been studied have apparently developed rather systematic approaches to the reproduction of adult target words.[2]

---

[2]Sometimes a particular word does seem to evoke an unsystematic series of potshots, and the difference between these words and others can be very striking. Ferguson and Farwell (1975) recorded a little girl's repeated attempts to say the word *pen* over the course of half an hour; they included the forms [mã͏ə], [dɛdn], [hɪn], [mbõ], [pɪn], [tntntn], [bah], [dʰaum], and [buã]. (Transcription is simplified from the original; raised symbols indicate weak sounds, and the tilde [˜] over a vowel indicates a nasalized pronunciation.)

Table 3.3   **Examples of Early Pronunciations of Common Words**

	Jacob (approx. 19 months)	Hildegard (approx. 24 months)	Daniel (approx. 25 months)	Amahl (A) (approx. 25 months)	Amahl (B) (approx. 32 months)
apple /æpl/	æpw	ʔapa	æpu[1]	ɛbu	æpəl
bottle /badl/	gʌgʌ	balu	baw	bɔgu	bɔkəl
water /wɔdr/[2]	—	walu	ɔərs	wɔːdə	wɔːtə
house /hæws/	—	haws	æws	aut	haut
dog/doggie /dɔg/ /dɔgi/	dadi	doti	gɔg	gɔgi	dɔg
cookie /kuki/	kikʌ kʌki	tuti	guki	—	—
shoe /ʃu/	du ʃɪw	ʒu	u	duː	tuː
sock /sak/	sʌk	—	ak	gɔk	tɔk
stone /ston/	—	doɪʃ	non	duːn	—

Note: ʔ is the glottal closure phone heard between the syllables of the expression "uh-oh" /ʌʔow/.
  ː indicates lengthening of preceding vowel.

[1]Young children sometimes pronounce the vowels [u] and [o] without the [w] "off-glide" characteristic of adult pronunciation.

[2]Amahl's model was British "Received Pronunciation" /wɔtə/.

Source: Amahl's data in this chapter are from Smith, 1973; Hildegard's are from Leopold, 1970, and may also be found in Moskowitz, 1970.

Feature Changes

For most children's early speech we can find a core of words that show very clear patterns. Let us begin with two hypothetical examples, simplified for the sake of clarity. One might find a child who gives these pronunciations:

Child A

pot [bat] ("bot")	back [bæk] (correct)
top [dap] ("dop")	day [dej] (correct)
cat [gæt] ("gat")	game [gejm] (correct)

Child A seems to use voiced stops in word-initial position both when they are appropriate (in the righthand column) and when the corresponding unvoiced stop is required (in the lefthand column). The place of articulation in all of these words is correct, however.

Another hypothetical child might pronounce the same words this way:

Child B

pot [pat] (correct)	back [bæt] ("bat")
top [tap] (correct)	day [dej] (correct)
cat [tæt] ("tat")	game [dejm] ("dame")

Child B has voicing correct but is unable to manage the velar place of articulation; attempts at adult words containing /k/ come up with a [t] instead, and a [d] for /g/.

These hypothetical examples make it clear that there are two important benefits to be derived from descriptions in terms of features as well as in terms of segments. First, instead of saying that the child uses this sound instead of that one, we can see that the child's attempt may be partly right and partly wrong. For example, hypothetical Child A gets position of articulation right but voicing wrong for unvoiced stops. Children in general get things partly right before they get them correct, so it is valuable to have a way of describing their attempts that deals with some of the attributes of a segment individually. In fact, even features can prove to be too crude a tool for some needs, as we shall see.

The second benefit of using features is that it allows one to see what several different-looking errors may have in common. Using a feature description, it is evident that the three mistakes of Child A were essentially identical. All were errors in which word-initial unvoiced stops were replaced by voiced stops. Similarly, the three mistakes of Child B were all a case of using an alveolar articulation when the target word required a velar. Patterns or families of errors like this are very common in child language (and also in second language acquisition).

Patterns are not always so regular, however. Sometimes a child may learn to get voicing correct for, say, /t/ and /d/, and yet still use [b] for /p/; another child may follow the general pattern of using voiced stops for unvoiced stops at the beginnings of words but have one or two words in which a word-initial /t/ appears to be produced correctly. An adequate theory of the acquisition of phonology must be able to accommodate both the regular and irregular relations between the child's attempt and the target word. We can thus rule out theories that try to describe the acquisition of phonology only in terms of the acquisition of features. The individual phonemes, and even individual words, often must be taken into account.

Cluster Reductions

Let's consider some other typical patterns of early pronunciation. Sequences of two consonants, or consonant clusters, appear to cause problems for most young speakers, and there are several patterns that children follow in dealing with them. Many children simply leave out one of the sounds. In English /s/ + stop consonant clusters are very common, and children often omit the /s/. Daniel, for example, would have produced the forms given in the first column of examples.

	Daniel	Stephen
spill	[pɪl] ("pill")	[fɪl] ("fill")
store	[tɔr] ("tore")	[sɔr] ("sore")
school	[kul] ("cool")	[sul] ("sool")

A less-common pattern, found perhaps in 10 percent of children learning English, is to leave out the stop consonant, as we see in the treatment of *store* and *school* in the second column. Frequently, the children like Stephen, who omit alveolar and velar stops in these clusters, do something a little different with /sp/ clusters. They use [f], not /s/. This [f] appears to be an attempt to match the sound of the whole cluster within a single consonant. It has the fricative character of the /s/ but the labial character of the /p/. (English has no bilabial fricative; the labiodental /f/ is the closest a child can come to the bilabial fricative sound [ɸ] unless he teaches himself to make a segment that he has never heard, and some children do just this, using [ɸ] for /sp/ and also the non-English velar fricative [x] for /sk/.)

Other kinds of clusters may also be treated by omission of one of the sounds, as in column 1 of the example that follows. However, these stop + liquid clusters are sometimes broken up by an unstressed vowel, as in column 2. We also find the use of [w] for the liquid, as in column 3.

	1	2	3
bread	[bɛd] ("bed")	[bərɛ́d] ("buh-RED")	[bwɛd] ("bwed")
blue	[bu] ("boo")	[bəlu´] ("buh-LOO")	[bwu] ("bwoo")

Writing Rules

We can write down abbreviated, explicit statements for regular patterns of correspondence between child and adult sound patterns when they occur; such statements are usually called *child phonology* rules. Rules become particularly useful when we are trying to understand a child's form in which several different correspondence patterns are superimposed. For example, a child who has a pattern or rule of replacing velar stops with alveolars and another rule of approximating initial /sp/ with [f] would probably say the word *speak* as [fit] ("feet"); two separate rules have been applied independently.

Accuracy of Perception

Sometimes it is suggested that children who fail to pronounce particular sounds correctly have failed to perceive them accurately. Wholesale confusion of two similar adult phonemes may happen. Children learning English do appear to have some problems distinguishing between words that begin with a few pairs of extremely similar sounds, such as [f] and [θ], and this may contribute to the generally late acquisition of [θ] (Velleman, 1988). But usually, children with normal hearing are able to perform such discrimination tasks quite well, provided they are thoroughly familiar with both test words in a pair (Barton, 1980). Hence, hypothetical Child A described earlier might well be able to point correctly to a coat and a goat even while calling them both "goat."

Although complete fusion of two similar adult phonemes appears to be relatively uncommon for children who have begun to speak, misidentification of one segment in an individual word is reported to occur quite frequently (Macken, 1980; see also Butler Platt & MacWhinney, 1983). This is usually discovered in the following way: A child who has been producing [f] for both /f/ and /s/ at last begins to get an [s]-like sound for almost all adult words that begin with /s/, including those that she used to say with [f]. However, there are still one or two words that begin with /s/ that she continues to pronounce with the old [f]. The usual explanation of this phenomenon is that in those one or two lagging words, the child had misidentified the initial segments; she really thought they began with /f/, either on first hearing them or after listening to her own erroneous renditions.

Suprasegmental–Segmental Interactions

In the early period of development, word pronunciations are often affected by length of the **word and stress patterns.** For example, it is quite common for young children to omit the initial syllable of a multisyllabic word when that syllable is unstressed. Thus, we have forms like "mato" for *tomato,* "zert" for *dessert,* and "posed" for *supposed.* Unstressed syllables in medial position may also be omitted in words like *telephone* [tɛfon] and *elephant* [ɛfənt]. In final position, however, it is much less common for unstressed syllables to be omitted.

Pronunciations of this type do not appear to be due to difficulties with production of particular sounds, but rather to problems with the stress patterns of the words. Since weakly stressed syllables are harder to perceive, the errors may be due to perception rather than production. However, since final unstressed syllables are usually not omitted, most such perceptual problems cannot simply be a matter of not hearing the unstressed syllable; they must instead have to do with selective attention—perhaps the child who makes such errors only "tunes in" to the word when the stressed syllable starts. Another pattern is found in children who use **dummy syllables,** such as [tə] or [rɪ], to take the place of many or all initial unstressed syllables (Smith, 1973). Obviously, in such cases the child knows that the initial unstressed syllable is present. In some instances, perhaps his knowledge of the sounds in the adult syllable may be incomplete; in others, the problem may be organizing the production of the sounds using this less-common stress pattern. Suprasegmental patterns are also involved in the acquisition of grammatical morphemes (see Gerken & McIntosh, 1993; Peters & Menn, 1993).

Assimilation

So far we have talked about the ways in which children approximate the sounds of segments or clusters. However, in recent years we have come to understand that many of the ways in which children adapt adult words cannot be explained without taking the sounds of the whole target word into account. Daniel (Menn, 1971) showed the following pattern:

- Initial voiced stops usually showed correct position of stop articulation and correct voicing.

  Set 1

bump	[bʌmp]	(correct)
down	[dæwn]	(correct)
gone	[gɔn]	(correct)

- Initial unvoiced stops usually showed correct position but incorrect voicing.

  Set 2

pipe	[bajp]	("bipe")
toad	[dowd]	("dode")
car	[gar]	("gar")

However, when Daniel attempted to say a word that begins with a stop in one place of articulation and ends with a stop in a different place of articulation, a very striking kind of error occurred:

- Initial labial stops became [g] when the target word ended with a velar stop.

  Set 3

bug	[gʌg]	("gug")
big	[gɪg]	("gig")
book	[guk]	("gook")
bike	[gajk]	("gike")
pig	[gɪg]	("gig")

- Initial alveolar stops and *s* + stop clusters also became [g] when the target word ended with a velar stop.

  Set 4

dog	[gɔg]	("gawg")
Doug	[gʌg]	("gug")
duck	[gʌk]	("guck")
stick	[gɪk]	("gick")

- Initial alveolar stops and *s* + stop clusters became [b] when the target word ended with a labial stop.

Set 5

tub	[bʌb]	("bub")
top	[bap]	("bop")
step	[bɛp]	("bep")
stop	[bap]	("bop")

We cannot explain Daniel's changes in the initial consonants as an inability to pronounce the stops since he was able to get all three places of articulation correct individually (i.e., when there was only one stop in a word or two stops that shared the same place of articulation, as in *bump* or *pipe* in sets 1 and 2). However, when an adult word contained two stops with different places of articulation, he could only get one of the places right, and the place of the other stop was changed to match.

A change in one sound to make it more like another is called **assimilation.** (An example of nasal assimilation was given on p. 90–91) One can see how rapidly a simple assimilation pattern like this one renders a child unintelligible to a person who is not familiar with the child's speech. Who would know that to decode *gig*, one must consider whether the context called for *big, pig,* or *dig?* And of course, there are many frustrating times when such a child's utterances remain unintelligible because the context does not give enough cues.

Assimilation may also involve manner rather than place of articulation, with similar effects on intelligibility. As was mentioned in the section on regression, Daniel later made initial consonants nasal if the final consonant or consonant cluster contained a nasal.

bump	[mʌmp]	("mump")
beans	[minz]	("means")
dance	[næns]	("nance")
going	[ŋowɪŋ]	(cannot be spelled with English orthography)

Examples like these make it clear that tests or speech samples used for study of articulation must consider all the sounds in a target word. It would have been incorrect to say that Daniel, at either of the two stages just described, could not pronounce word-initial /b/ or /d/, which one might conclude from looking at his versions of *big, dog, duck, beans,* and *dance.* It is very important to use words with only one position and one manner of stop articulation—like *pipe, bib, daddy, papa, do, go, cake*—to assess stop production. Texts on functional articulation disorders (phonological disability) in children (Grunwell, 1987; Ingram, 1989; Stoel-Gammon & Dunn, 1985) make this point clearly. This quite normal two-year-old child's problem was in managing certain sound sequences, not in articulating the sounds themselves.

Rule Origin

Discovery of Rules

We have seen that many children have regular ways of replacing sounds in adult words; and if there is a regularity, we can write a rule to describe it. If the child has mastered accurate productions of adult sounds, these are also to be counted among the child's regularities, and rules (trivial-sounding but often useful) like "adult /t/ becomes child [t]" can be written for them as well.

So far, we have discussed several error patterns that are regular enough to be abbreviated as rules: for example, a rule making all initial stops voiced (hypothetical Child A), a rule replacing all velar stops by alveolar ones (hypothetical Child B), a rule omitting [s] in word-initial consonant clusters, a rule changing initial stops to nasals if there is a nasal at the end of the word, and a more complex pattern involving rules of velar and labial assimilation (Menn, 1971). In general, it appears to be the case, as common sense would suggest, that children produce these patterns because they cannot yet produce any more accurate match to the adult target sound or sound sequence (except perhaps transiently during imitation). There are exceptions to this common-sense view, however; a child who has finally learned to say a sound or sound sequence in some new words may continue in her habit of changing that sound or sequence to something else in old words and in new words that very closely resemble the old words. Rules, once acquired, appear to have a life of their own.

Many phonological error patterns that children use can be explained as fairly natural outcomes of imperfectly coordinated articulatory movements. For example, trouble in delaying the start of vocal cord vibration after the release of a stop would mean a tendency to produce all stops as voiced. The assorted errors that we see in early attempts at producing consonant clusters could be due to various ways of compensating for trouble in producing rapid shifts in manner and/or place of articulation. Such natural error patterns and the rules describing them are usually referred to as **natural processes** (Edwards & Shriberg, 1983; Ingram, 1989). However, individual children sometimes have error patterns which do not seem very "natural," such as use of [h] for a large number of different adult consonants.

Error patterns in a child's first handful of words are often not regular enough for rule writing. Early words typically include a few (progressive) phonological idioms and also a few grossly variable and inaccurate forms (e.g., "bye-bye" produced as [bæ-bæ], [ga-ga], and [ɣæ-ɣæ]; the symbol [ɣ] (gamma) denotes a voiced velar fricative. Apparently it generally takes a child some time to develop regular ways—accurate or inaccurate—of dealing with adult sounds. This suggests that rules, even natural ones, are discovered by trial and error rather than coming into play automatically as the child starts to speak. This view is basic to the cognitive problem-solving approach to developmental phonology, but it is at odds with the most strongly nativist versions of

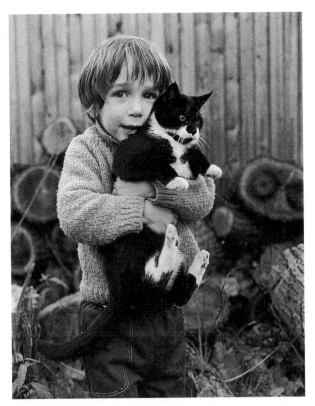

Assimilation leads this child to say "tat."

the "natural phonology" approach, which predict that natural processes will operate most generally at the beginning of speech and then gradually be overcome (e.g., Stampe, 1969).

Canonical Forms

We concluded earlier that children learn sound sequences, not just sounds. The beginning speaker appears to discover how to say certain word-length sequences of sounds and then to attempt similar approaches to other adult words that he perceives as being similar to his initial conquests. In cognitive terms the solution of a problem—how to say a particular word—is generalized to similar problems. This procedure, first described in exquisite detail in a diary study by Waterson (1971), results in the development of little groups of words; each group consists of the child's renditions of adult words that are somewhat similar and have usually become even more similar in the child's versions. Consider the following sets of words from Waterson's work:

Set 1		Set 2	
Randall	[ɲaɲo]	fish	[ɪʃ]
window	[ɲeːɲeː]	dish	[dɪʃ]
finger	[ɲeːɲeː] or [ɲiːɲɪ]	vest	[uʃ]
another	[ɲaɲa]	brush	[byʃ]
		fetch	[ɪʃ]

Note. [ɲ] represents a palatal nasal, roughly the sound of *ny* in *canyon*.

[e] is used without [j] "off-glide."

[y] is the front rounded vowel spelled *u* in French and *ü* in German.

: indicates that the preceding phone was of relatively long duration.

Each little group can be described by abstracting out what the child's renditions have in common. The words in the first column are disyllables consisting of two palatal nasals [ɲ] and two vowels. The words in the second column all end with the palatal fricative [ʃ], contain a short vowel made with the tongue relatively high in the mouth, and begin with either a stop or that vowel. Using V to stand for any vowel and C to stand for any stop consonant, we can abbreviate the two patterns just presented; the first is [ɲVɲV], and the second is [(C)Vʃ]. (Putting the C in parentheses is a standard way of indicating that it is sometimes omitted.)

Such abstracted patterns for sets of words are called **canonical forms,** and each word that conforms to that pattern is then an instance of that canonical form. The output of children who have more than about five but fewer than perhaps a hundred words can generally be described as several sets of canonical forms plus a handful of other words, usually phonological idioms, that are relatively isolated.

This organization of children's early vocabulary is currently seen as the key to understanding most of their ways of dealing with adult words. A child's canonical forms represent the kinds of sound sequences that she has learned to produce at will up to that point; her rules are representations of the regular ways that she adjusts adult words to fit into those available sequences. Not all children arrive at regular ways to make these adjustments; Daniel did but Waterson's subject did not, and neither did the children reported by Macken (1979) and Priestly (1977).

Children who do use rules may start to do so at different points in their development. Some researchers distinguish a prerule period, "the stage of the first fifty words," from a later rule-governed period, but we must be careful to bear in mind the great amount of individual variation across children and the fact that some aspects of a child's phonology can be quite rule-governed while other aspects remain irregular.

Instrumental Analyses of Children's Speech

An unanswered question thus far is whether the transcriber's ear is fully adequate to evaluate children's speech. We have described children's words with the same symbols that we use for adult phones and phonemes, but is this use really justified? Macken and Barton (1980) have shown that some degree of caution is necessary in transcribing a child's speech on the basis of adult perceptions. Some children who appear to be using voiced stops for initial unvoiced stops are actually trying to make the correct distinction, but they have not learned to do so in a way that is audible to the unaided ear. Their use of longer voicing onset timing for their unvoiced stops than for their voiced ones is detectable only by laboratory measurements of the sound waves they produce. This is a case where a description of the child's language in terms of features is too crude to give an accurate reflection of what is happening. A child who is making an inaudible but correct distinction between voiced and unvoiced stops has the correct phonological distinction but an inadequate version of the phonetic distinction; it would not be correct to describe him either as having mastered or as not having understood the voicing distinction for initial stops. He is at an intermediate stage.

Strategies in Learning to Pronounce

A major focus of research in child phonology, as in developmental psychology, has been the study of differences among children. The data presented so far have shown several differences in the rules describing the forms that various children use. If we look at the overall strategies that children adopt to deal with the problem of producing words, another type of difference becomes apparent. Some children might be thought of as relatively conservative; they seem not to use a word if they cannot produce at least the beginning sounds fairly accurately. In a list of the words such a child recognizes compared to the words she uses, there may be a very striking imbalance; for example, Jacob, who has been cited several times in this chapter, understood and responded to many words beginning with /b/, /k/, and /d/ but only attempted to say those be with /d/ (with the exception of "bye-bye," which he said under social pressure and which came out [da-da]). This state of affairs lasted for several months; then a group of /k/-initial words were observed, all produced with a correct first segment, and then initial /b/ was finally mastered.

Clearly, Jacob was sticking to what he knew how to pronounce and avoiding other words until he had figured out how to produce them to his own satisfaction. Other children have also been observed to avoid certain sounds (Ferguson & Farwell, 1975), although until quite recently few people thought it was possible for a child of, say, fifteen months to have such a degree of phonological awareness. This skepticism was reinforced by the fact that many other children, often two years old or older, seem blissfully unaware of the discrepancy between what they are saying and the adult target. Most children probably fall between the extremes of selecting only what they can say, on the one hand, and casually adapting any adult word to fit their output repertoire on the other hand (see Schwartz & Leonard, 1982).

Another dimension of acquisition strategy seems closely related to Katherine Nelson's (1973) referential/expressive dimension (see Chapters 4 and 8). Some children attempt one word at a time, and these words generally have relatively clear and consistent (although possibly quite incorrect) pronunciation. Others use a more global approach to speech, approximating whole phrases with much less clear or consistent articulation (Branigan, 1979; Peters, 1977). The child's meaning may be understandable from context and tone of voice, and there may be enough recognizable phonetic material in the utterance to make it clear that particular words are intended; yet the phrase may be reduced to a virtually untranscribable mess.

There are other children who combine these approaches; for example, some embed one or two clear words in long, otherwise unintelligible strings. We know very little about why such differences among children exist or whether they correlate with any other developmental phenomena. However, as the selectors and the adaptors learn more sounds and as the one-worders start to put words together and the phrase-approximators become more precise in their articulation, the distinctions in strategy eventually blur and seem to disappear.

Change over Time: The Increasing Importance of Child-Phonology Rules

Let's review the developmental changes that we have seen up to now. A child's acquisition of phonology begins with trial-and-error attempts at isolated words, especially ones that match her favorite babble patterns. Some of these may be produced quite accurately, and these will become notable as progressive phonological idioms; others may be very loosely and variably approximated. Eventually, the child will be able to generalize some of his successes; thus, little groups of similar-sounding words form in his output repertoire. Canonical forms can be written to describe what the words in each group have in common; these help to capture the severe restrictions on what sounds can co-occur in the child's output.

A way of dealing with a group of adult words may be extended to a similar word that the child has already been pronouncing; if the old form was a closer approximation to the adult model than the new one, the change is a regressive one, as in Daniel's change from "down" to "noun" described earlier. If the adult words have regular correspondences to the child's words, rules can be written abstracting those regularities, and regression will be appropriately considered as a case of rule overgeneralization. This is the picture that we have described up to this point.

Now, gradually, an important change occurs. The child becomes able to combine a greater variety of sounds in a word. He no longer appears to be operating with little families of similar words but with segments, and so description in terms of canonical forms loses its usefulness. In psycholinguistic terms this development would reflect the ability to analyze a perceived word into segments and to pronounce those segments relatively independently. This development toward word segmentation is never complete, even in an adult, but the child moves toward whatever degree of combinatorial freedom the surrounding adults possess.

The developing ability to deal with individual segments increases the value of writing explicit rules to describe the child's renditions of those segments. N. V. Smith's child Amahl (Smith, 1973) gives a splendid example of this level of developing ability, and we will conclude this section with an account of his development of an initial [tʃ] ("ch"). This portion of Smith's study is particularly interesting because it shows that one needs to consider the range of variation in a child's renditions of adult segments in order to decide which ones the child is treating as "the same" and which ones she is treating as distinct. The clinical and research importance of this example cannot be overemphasized; several elicitations of each test word are required to establish a child's ways of rendering the sounds in it. Gradual replacement of one way of saying a word with a new way of saying it, as illustrated here, is the norm, not the exception. However, if only a single sample of a word is obtained in a given observation, these orderly but gradual changes can be mistaken for wildly random variation.

At a certain point late in his second year, referred to as stage 19 in Smith's (1973) book, Amahl used a *t*-like phone correctly for the stop /t/ and incorrectly for the fricative /s/ and the affricate stop /tʃ/. The following data are taken (in simplified notation) from a table that summarizes the changes in the renditions of three words beginning with these sounds (p. 154).

Target:	toe	say	chair
	/tow/	/sej/	[tʃeʌ]
Output:			
Stage 19	[to]	[tej]	[teʌ]
20	[to]	[tej], [tsej]	[teʌ], [tseʌ]
21	[to]	[tsej], [sej]	[tseʌ], [seʌ]
22	[to]	[sej]	[seʌ]
26	[to]	[sej]	[seʌ], [tseʌ]
29	[to]	[sej]	[tseʌ]
			[tʃeʌ]

Note: The target dialect, British "Received Pronunciation," has no [r] in word-final position.

We see that Amahl said these three beginning sounds all as [t] at stage 19. At stage 20, however, he had separated the target /t/ from the other sounds and had begun to use [ts] for the friction sounds of /s/ and /tʃ/ in some productions of *say* and *chair*. He was at this point capable of *making* the output distinction between /t/ and the other two sounds but not of *maintaining* it.

At stage 21 he had clearly severed the connection of /s/ and /tʃ/ with /t/; for now the friction sound was always present in his renditions of the first two sounds. However, it becomes increasingly clear that as far as output is concerned, there is no distinction between /s/ and /tʃ/, for the sound [s] is appearing for both of these. By stage 22 and for the next three stages (not shown), [s] is used reliably for them both. Note that although this is fine for the true /s/ sound, it is an overcorrection for the target /tʃ/; [ts] was a more accurate rendition of this sound.

Finally, at stage 26 Amahl's productions start to represent the phonemic distinction between /s/ and /tʃ/; he starts to use [ts] again in *chair,* and by stage 29 the use of [s] for /tʃ/ has disappeared. The final phonetic detail of replacing the [ts] (which we may consider an alveolar affricate) with the palatal affricate /tʃ/ comes later.

Development after Three Years

Although children's pronunciation patterns are not fully adultlike by three years of age, the basic features of the adult phonological system are present. Studies of groups of children tested at different ages (e.g., Prather, Hedrick, & Kern, 1975; Templin, 1957) provide a general picture of the acquisition of English during the period of *mas-*

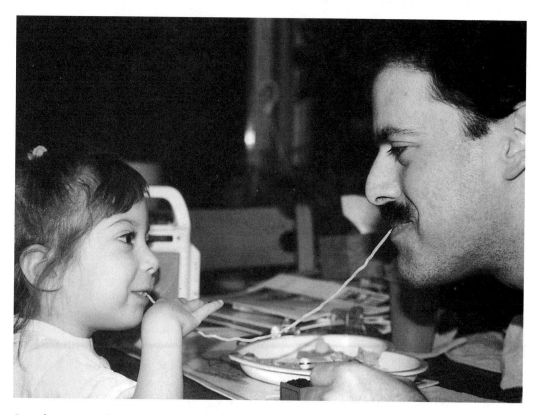

Initial consonant clusters can make a word like "spaghetti" difficult for preschoolers to pronounce.

tery. These studies are important because they provide guidelines that speech therapists can use in identifying children whose phonological system is not developing normally (see Chapter 9). By three, most children can produce all the vowel sounds and nearly all the consonant sounds. This does not mean that their productions are 100 percent accurate, but rather that the sounds are produced correctly in at least a few words. Consonants that are likely to be in error, even at the age of four or five, are the liquids /r/ and /l/ and the fricatives /v/, /θ/ as in *thin,* and /ð/ as in *the.* As might be expected, correct pronunciation patterns are often more accurate in short words, like the /v/ of *vase,* while longer words like *vacuum cleaner* may cause mispronunciations. In most cases, correct production of all sounds is achieved by around seven years of age.

Consonant clusters such as [spr-] at the beginning of the word *spring* and [-lps] at the end of *helps* are usually acquired relatively late. In some cases, the child is capable of producing the individual phonemes within the cluster, but not of putting them together in a sequence. Thus, the /s/ of *see* and the /n/ of *no* could be pronounced correctly whereas the /sn-/ combination in *snow* would be produced with omission of the /s/. (Examples of this pattern of "cluster of reduction" were presented earlier; see page 96). Smit and colleagues (Smit, 1993; Smit et al., 1990) report that some clusters in word-initial position are not mastered until the age of seven or eight years.

The Acquisition of English Morphophonology

Children begin learning some of the regularities governing the choice among English allomorphs fairly early. However, some aspects of English stress appear not to be mastered until age twelve or so, and some nonproductive regularities are still being learned well into adolescence. Much work remains to be done in this area, but we will discuss two pioneering experimental studies.

Myerson (1975) carried out a study that showed an increasing ability over the ages eight through seventeen to deal with three types of allomorphy: (1) the change from alveolar stop to palatal fricative when *-ion* is added, as in *explode–explosion;* (2) the shift in stress when *-ity* or *-ical* are added to words like *stupid (stupidity)* or *method (methodical);* and (3) the changes in vowels associated with such shifts in stress.

It had been known for some time (Krohn, Steinberg, & Kobayashi, 1972) that adults do not reliably make these changes in consonants, stress, and vowels when they are simply asked to tack on endings like *-ion* or *-ity* to nonsense words or to existing words that do not occur with these endings. This situation holds true for children as well. However, Myerson showed that older children and adolescents do gradually learn to make use of these relationships, which apparently reduce the load on long-term memory storage of words. Myerson taught seventy-two children (eighteen each from grades 3, 6, 9, and 12) ten pairs of made-up words presented as meaningful. Each subject was presented with the same base "word" and one of two versions of that base word with an ending (-*ion*, -*ical*, or -*ity*) attached. One of those two versions followed an English pattern; for example, a base that rhymed with *distort* was paired with a derived form rhyming with *distortion*. The other version of the derived form just tacked the ending onto the base without change so that the subject was taught a base rhyming with *distort,* and a derived form that was pronounced "distortean" (rather like what one would call a native of a place called Distortea). Each subject learned five pairs of words made up according to the English pattern and five pairs of words with the same endings just tacked on. The pairs were thoroughly taught in the first session and then tested for recall one day, one week, and six weeks later. The teaching procedure went according to the following example:

> A picture of a lion about to pounce on a pig is presented while the following paragraph is read aloud: "*Delort.* To delort means to attack. The lion is about to delort the pig. The lion is about to attack the pig. Now add *i-o-n* to *delort* to make a new word meaning an attack. The lion is about to delort the pig. Whenever a lion delorts a pig, he makes a (*version 1*) /dəlɔrtiʌn/ (*version 2*) /dəlorʒn/. What does a lion do when he delorts a pig? He makes a _____. Whenever a lion delorts a pig, he makes a _____." Any errors are corrected. (Appendix p. xxix)

Similar presentations were used for pairs like *glane–glanity* (/gléjnəti/, /glǽnəti/) and *gathod–gathodical* (/ˈgǽθədɪkl/, /gəˈθádɪkl/).

Myerson found that the forms with the tacked-on endings were harder to recall for all children. Furthermore, there was an overwhelming tendency for a child who had been taught a tacked-on form like *delortean* to recall it incorrectly as *delortion,* a form that had the appropriate allomorphic base change, whereas the opposite error of recalling a *delortion* form as *delortean* rarely occurred.

Atkinson-King (1973) also studied an aspect of word stress, the acquisition of the word-stress difference that distinguishes the noun *record* from the verb *record.* She found that kindergartners, the youngest children in her study, were able to listen to pairs of sentences like "I put the record (/rékrd/) on the shelf" and "I put the record (/rekɔ́rd/) on the shelf" and judge correctly that the first was better. They were also able to produce emphatic stress correctly, as in "I want the réd book, not the green book." The major portion of her study, however, was a large set of imitation, judgment, and production tests of children's ability to distinguish phrases like "a green hóuse" or "the red sócks" from compounds like "a gréenhouse" or "the Réd Sox" (the name of the baseball team from Boston, where the study was carried out).

For example, in one test the children were given pairs of pictures and asked to show which was the greenhouse and which was the green house. In a second task the children were given pairs of sentences, such as "I put mustard on my hót dog" and "I put mustard on my hot dóg," and asked which one was better. In a third task the children were given the pictures singly and asked to label them; adults heard tapes of their productions and attempted to decide which of the pair each child had intended. In a fourth test the children were given the pair of pictures together and asked to describe them so that the investigator could tell which was which. This one gave some curious results, for Atkinson-King found that

> some children knew that there was a difference between members of a pair but could not consistently and correctly signal that difference. For example, some used the same stress pattern on both members of a pair but said the entire first member very rapidly and the second extremely slowly (in this presentation, half the time the first member of the pair was the phrase and half the time it was the compound). A number of others were able to produce the two stress patterns correctly but always produced the compound and then the phrasal pattern, regardless of the order in which the pictures they were looking at appeared. (p. 111)

Note that this confusion did not indicate a general inability to control stress, since all of the children had been shown able to produce emphatic stress accurately.

All the children, even the kindergartners, could imitate each pair accurately, but the ability to deal with the other tasks at an adult level of performance (essentially perfect) developed gradually from first grade to sixth grade. Preference judgments were 80 percent correct by third grade; the ability to choose between two pictures given the label for one of them was acquired next, then the ability to produce the two labels accurately when presented with the paired pictures, and finally the ability to produce the label distinguishably when given only one of the pictures. The first two tasks (imitation and preference) may be seen as testing phonetic ability—can the child get the sound right and know how it should sound in context? The others require the ability to make a choice between stress patterns without the support of linguistic context; this can be considered a phonemic skill.

Parental Role in Phonological Development

It is often said that overt correction by adults plays no role in the acquisition of language, at least with respect to phonology and syntax. Certainly it can fail to have any noticeable effect, and the arguments against external-reward behaviorist models of acquisition show that, in any case, the child's own self-monitoring, quite possibly taking place below the level of consciousness, must be responsible for the bulk of the acquisition of phonology. The general (but not total) resistance of phonological errors to overt correction appears to reflect the difficulty of modifying any aspect of habitual or automatic behavior, including slouching at the table and allowing the screen door to slam. Conscious efforts trickle down to automatic behavior slowly, if at all. Yet learning—in the case of phonology, incredibly precise learning—does take place over time; children adjust their production of words so that it approaches some composite of their parents and their peers (Deser, 1990; Payne, 1976).

They acquire the regional and stylistic variants that they hear—which of course has major clinical and research implications. We often cannot tell whether a child's form that differs from our own is correct or incorrect until we compare it with how the child's parents and/or slightly older friends would say the same word in the same setting. A child with parents from New York who pronounces *bang* as [bĭəŋg] or one from the West who says it as [beŋ] is just as correct as one from the Middle Atlantic who says [bæŋ]. We must not be misled by the fact that the last form matches the spelling of *bang* better; the child's target is the spoken word, not the written one.

Similarly, although young children are often given the opportunity to hear nouns in isolation in naming routines, they usually hear most other words in phrases, and the "targets" that they are trying to pronounce must be considered to be these phrasal forms (i.e., forms like *hafta, wan'em, couldja,* and so on).

Parents do seem to improve the precision of their articulation above normal conversational levels to help their children learn to speak, however. Two researchers, Malsheen (1980) and Bernstein Ratner (1984a, 1984b) have carried out major studies of this phenomenon using acoustic measurements to show that parents increase the articulatory precision of their speech to children in the first few years of their children's learning to speak. This adult behavior is probably not conscious either, except as an attempt to assure understanding; but there seems to be more to it than that, according to Bernstein Ratner.

Malsheen tape-recorded mothers of two children who had not yet produced any recognizable words (six and eight months old), two children who had produced one-word utterances (fifteen and sixteen months old), and two children (two-and-a-half and five years old) who had used an average of several words per utterance. She compared the word-initial consonants (*b, d, g, p, t, k*) used by each woman in speaking to her child and in speaking to an adult, and she found that mothers clarified their pronunciation of initial consonants in speech to the children at the one-word stage but not to the prelingual children or to the older ones. She measured this clarification in terms of the same parameter used by Macken and Barton, the voice onset time (the period between the release of the oral closure and the onset of vocal cord vibration). Recall that voiced word-initial stops in English are not necessarily produced with concurrent vocal cord vibration but that voicing begins, on the average, well within two hundredths of a second after the release of closure (when a vowel follows); in the production of unvoiced stops, vocal cord vibration usually begins more than four hundredths of a second after the release. However, in normal adult–adult conversation consonant production is quite sloppy; for example, in Malsheen's adult–adult conversations as many as half of the instances of word-initial /t/ had voice onset time of less than two hundredths of a second, which means that they would have been heard as /d/ if they had been taken out of context. The same kind of sloppy control was also found in the mothers' speech to the prelingual children and to the children who were using multiword utterances. However, speech to the children in the one-word stage showed very few sloppy unvoiced stops; almost all were produced with a voice onset time of four hundredths of a second or more, and many were hyper-distinct with voice onset time of over a tenth of a second.

Bernstein Ratner studied vowel production of nine mothers speaking to their children (some at the one-word stage and some using an average of two to four words per utterance) as compared with the vowels in the same words excerpted from speech to other adults. Her findings indicate that mothers' clarification of vowel production is best seen as modeling words of the type that the child is currently learning to use, rather than increasing the distinctness of overall speech. What she found was that speech directed to children at the one-word stage showed clarification of vowels in nouns, verbs, and adjectives—that is, the sort of words being used most by the children themselves. Speech directed to children using several-word utterances showed clarification not only in nouns, verbs, and adjectives, but also in the function words that these children were just beginning to use: pronouns, prepositions, and conjunctions.

Summary

Phonology concerns the relations among the speech sounds of a language: their phonetic resemblances due to the way they are produced, their distributions as shown by minimal-pair contrasts, the possible phonotactic sequences in which they occur, and the way that distinct phonemes correspond to one another in the several allomorphs that a morpheme can have. The child learning to talk must learn to produce the right sounds, to put them in the sequences demanded by the ambient language, to recognize variant phones as representative of the same phoneme, and to learn at least the productive allomorphic relationships.

Humans have an innate, biological basis for hearing and producing speech sounds; this is then shaped by language experience, including cognitive reactions to articulatory challenges. There is strong evidence to suggest that normal infants are born with the ability to hear many distinctions between speech sounds, but that around age ten to twelve months their auditory perceptions become adultlike—that is, they become less sensitive to those differences that are subphonemic in whatever language is around them. Infants also appear to progress through the early months of sound production in a biologically determined way, for the detrimental effects of deafness on production only start to appear after reduplicated babbling has begun. Individual differences and ambient language effects gradually appear in later babbling. The transition from babbling to speech is gradual; early words tend to utilize sounds that the child has been favoring in late babbling.

Nativist theories of phonological development emphasize the similarities among children; they have difficulty dealing with individual differences and with irregularities. In addition, the best-known nativist theory, that of Jakobson, deals only with the acquisition of phonemic contrast, not with phonetic targets or phonotactic patterns. Behaviorist theories that depend on external reward for improved pronunciation are inadequate; external reward is too crude to guide mastery of the myriad fine details of phonetics. Neither nativist nor behaviorist theories can deal with regression in accuracy of production; here, as elsewhere in language acquisition, the data require a cognitive problem-solving theory since only this type of theory predicts that there will be overgeneralizations.

With the aid of descriptive features, we can assess children's partial successes in pronunciation and see similarities linking their attempts at related sounds. Rendering all initial stops as voiced, using alveolar place of articulation for both alveolar and velar consonants, and assimilating nasality and/or place of articulation are common patterns in early child phonology, as are several varieties of cluster simplification. When such patterns occur regularly in a given child's speech, rules can be written to describe the relation between the adult word and the child's form, for both correct and incorrect renditions. Even when the adult–child correspondences are not regular enough to be called rules, early child words typically occur in little groups whose common properties can be abstracted and written in formulas called canonical forms. Often there are a few words whose pronunciation is much more adultlike than others; these isolated progressive phonological idioms do not, by definition, come under any of the child's canonical forms but are exceptions to the child's rules. They are usually among the child's earliest words; this supports the claim that rules for rendering adult words are discovered by the child through trial and error.

Not all of a child's progress is correctly assessed by the unaided ear; instrumental studies of tape recordings show that children's earliest steps toward mastering adult phonemic distinctions may be inaudible to adults.

Individual variation among children is found in the strategies they adopt as well as in their individual rules and canonical forms. Some children attempt whole phrases, others try words singly; some avoid (public) attempts at words they cannot pronounce, others rearrange adult words freely to fit them into their existing repertoire.

Eventually, as the child learns to put more different kinds of speech sounds together within one word, the small groups expand and merge; canonical forms become less useful as descriptors, while rules become more useful.

In the elementary school years, children learn to distinguish certain aspects of the English stress system, and in the later school years they become acquainted with some of the nonproductive relationships that prevail among words in the Latin-based portion of the English lexicon. These relationships strongly affect recall and presumably reduce the memory load required for learning new words.

Overt parental correction of pronunciation has perhaps the same effect on children as correction of any other habitual behavior. Yet mothers have been shown to increase the accuracy of their production of word-initial consonants just as children are learning to pronounce single words and to enhance the clarity of their vowels in content words during the same period. Furthermore, they later increase the clarity of function word production slightly, when their children are beginning to express the grammatical relations that adult grammar encodes in function words.

Key Words

acoustic phonetics
affricates
allomorph
alveolar
assimilation
behaviorist
canonical form
categorical perception
consonant
consonant clusters
diphthongized
dummy syllable
free variation
fricative
glide
glottal
glottal fricative
high amplitude sucking
interdental
intonation contour
labial
labiodental
liquid
minimal pair
modulated babble
monophthongs
morpheme
nasal stop
nativist
natural processes
nonreflexive

obstruents
palatal
phone
phoneme
phonotactics
productive
progressive phonological idioms
protoword
reduplicated babble
reflexive
regression
self-organizing system
semivowels
sociolinguistics
sound play
stem allomorphy
stress
unvoiced fricative
unvoiced stop
variegated babble
velar
velum
voiced
voiced affricate
voiced fricative
voiced stop
voiceless affricate
voice onset time
vowel
word and stress patterns

Suggested Projects

The first three activities are time-consuming and, if carried out in full detail, might well take several weeks to complete.

1. Tape-record the babbling or speech of a child between the ages of twelve and thirty months, keeping notes of the child's accompanying activities. As soon as possible after this session, transcribe the sounds the child made and try to classify them into the types of vocalizations discussed in the chapter: sound play, conversational babble, protowords, and words. What problems, if any, do you face in making these distinctions? What additional information do you need? Are there any utterances about which you could never be sure? Are there any utterances that are none of the above? If yes, what keeps them from fitting into each of the four major categories? What would you call them?

2. Find a child whose speech is somewhat intelligible but whose pronunciation of words is still babyish. Tape-record and transcribe a half-hour of the child's speech during a play session. (A good-quality tape recorder will be needed for the best results; it will also help if you can get the child to wear a good external lavaliere microphone.) Can you find regularities in the way the child renders adult words? If not, can you find canonical output forms that the child seems to rely on? Are any adult sounds or sequences of sounds especially variable in the way the child produces them? If you do find some regularities, write rules to describe them. Do these rules have exceptions? Are the forms of these exceptions closer to the adult word or farther from it?

3. If you have no access to a child of the appropriate age for activities 1 or 2, go over the examples presented in this chapter, and write explicit rules to describe what the child is doing to the adult words. Which rules can be written simply as "Adult (target) segment X becomes child (output) segment Y"? Which ones must also mention other sounds in the target word? Which ones must mention whether the sound in the adult word is in initial, medial, or final position? If you can't answer the last question from the small number of cases presented for a given real or hypothetical child in this chapter, give two formulations: a general one, assuming that what you see is broadly representative of what the child does, and a narrow one, allowing for the possibility that the child does something quite different if the segments are not in the given word position. Consider formulating your rules in terms of features or in terms of phonemes. For each rule indicate which mode of formulation is more helpful in understanding what the child is doing, and explain why.

4. Consider the development of /s/ and /tʃ/ by N. V. Smith's child, as described on pages 106–107. Suppose you had only one sample of each word per stage. Show

how you might get rather different ideas of what the child was doing, depending on which rendition of each word appeared in your data.

Suggested Readings

Barton, D. P. (1980). Phonemic perception in children. In G. Yeni-Komshian, J. F. Kavanagh, & C. A. Ferguson (Eds.), *Child phonology: Vol. 2. Perception.* New York: Academic Press.

Bloch, B., & Trager, G. L. (1942). *Outline of linguistic analysis.* Baltimore: Linguistic Society of America.

Braine, M. D. S. (1974). On what might constitute a learnable phonology. *Language, 50,* 270–299.

Clumeck, H. (1980). The acquisition of tone. In G. Yeni-Komshian, J. F. Kavanagh, & C. A. Ferguson (Eds.), *Child phonology. Vol. 1. Production.* New York: Academic Press.

Ferguson, C. A., & Farwell, C. B. (1975). Words and sounds in early language acquisition. *Language, 51,* 439–491.

Ferguson, C. A., & Macken, M. A. (1980). Phonological development in children's play and cognition. In K. E. Nelson (Ed.), *Children's Language* (Vol. 4). New York: Gardner Press.

Ferguson, C. A., Menn, L., & Stoel-Gammon, C. (Eds.). (1992). *Phonological development: Models, research, implications.* Parkton, MD: York Press.

Fey, M., & Gandour, J. (1982). Rule discovery in early phonology acquisition. *Journal of Child Development, 9,* 71–82.

Grunwell, P. (1982). *Clinical phonology.* London: Croom Helm.

Grunwell, P. (1987). *The nature of phonological disability in children* (2nd ed.). London: Academic Press.

Halliday, M. A. K. (1975). *Learning how to mean: Explorations in the development of language.* London: Edward Arnold.

Hyman, L. M. (1975). *Phonology: Theory and analysis.* New York: Holt, Rinehart & Winston.

Ingram, D. (1986). Phonological patterns in the speech of young children. In P. Fletcher & M. Garman (Eds.), *Language acquisition* (2nd ed.). Cambridge, UK: Cambridge University Press.

Ingram, D. (1989). *Phonological disabilities in children.* London: Cole and Whurr.

Jakobson, R. (1968). *Child language, aphasia, and phonological universals* (A. Keiler, Trans.). The Hague: Mouton (first published 1941).

Jusczyk, P. W. (1992). Developing phonological categories for the speech signal. In Ferguson, C. A., Menn, L., & Stoel-Gammon, C. (Eds.), *Phonological development: Models, research, implications.* Parkton, MD: York Press.

Kent, R. D. (1992). The biology of phonological development. In Ferguson, C. A., Menn, L., & Stoel-Gammon, C. (Eds.), *Phonological development: Models, research, implications.* Parkton, MD: York Press.

Labov, William. (1972). *Sociolinguistic patterns.* Philadelphia: University of Pennsylvania Press.

Ladefoged, P. (1971). *A course in phonetics.* New York: Harcourt Brace Jovanovich.

Leonard, L. B., Newhoff, M., & Mesalam, L. (1980). Individual differences in early child phonology. *Applied Psycholinguistics, 1,* 7–30.

Leonard, L. B., Schwartz, R., Folger, M. K., & Wilcox, M. J. (1978). Some aspects of child phonology in imitative and spontaneous speech. *Journal of Child Language, 5,* 403–416.

Lindblom, B. (1992). Phonological units as adaptive emergents of lexical development. In Ferguson, C. A., Menn, L., & Stoel-Gammon, C. (Eds.), *Phonological development. Models, research, implications.* Parkton, MD: York Press.

Locke, J. L. (1983). *Phonological acquisition and change.* New York: Academic Press.

Macken, M. A. (1979). Developmental reorganization of phonology: A hierarchy of basic units of acquisition. *Lingua, 49,* 11–49.

Macken, M. A., & Barton, D. (1980). The acquisition of the voicing contrast in English: A study of voice onset time in word-initial stop consonants. *Journal of Child Language, 7,* 41–75.

Macken, M. A., & Ferguson, C. A. (1982). Cognitive aspects of phonological development: Model, evidence, and issues. In K. E. Nelson (Ed.), *Children's language* (Vol. 4). New York: Gardner Press.

MacNeilage, P., & Davis, B. (1990). Acquisition of speech production: The achievement of segmental independence. In W. J. Hardcastle & A. Marchal (Eds.), *Speech production and speech modelling.* Dordrecht: Kluwer Press.

MacWhinney, B. (1978). The acquisition of morphophonology. *Monographs of the Society for Research in Child Development, 43,* 1–2.

Malsheen, B. (1980). Two hypotheses for phonetic clarification in the speech of mothers to children. In G. Yeni-Komshian, J. F. Kavanagh, & C. A. Ferguson (Eds.), *Child phonology: Vol. 2. Perception.* New York: Academic Press.

Menn, L. (1983). Development of articulatory, phonetic, and phonological capabilities. In B. Butterworth (Ed.), *Language production* (Vol. 2). London: Academic Press.

Menyuk, P., Menn, L., & Silber, R. (1986). Early strategies for the perception and production of words and sounds. In P. Fletcher & M. Garman (Eds.), *Language acquisition* (2nd ed.). Cambridge, UK: Cambridge University Press.

Oller, D. K. (1980). The emergence of the sounds of speech in infancy. In G. Yeni-Komshian, J. F. Kavanagh, & C. A. Ferguson (Eds.), *Child phonology: Vol. 1. Production.* New York: Academic Press.

Painter, C. (1984). *Into the mother tongue: A case study in early language development.* London: Frances Pinter.

Peters, A. M. (1977). Language learning strategies. *Language, 53,* 560–573.

Peters, A. M. (1983). *The units of language acquisition.* Cambridge, UK: Cambridge University Press.

Priestly, T. M. S. (1977). One idiosyncratic strategy in the acquisition of phonology. *Journal of Child Language, 4,* 45–66.

Smith, N. V. (1973). *The acquisition of phonology: A case study.* Cambridge, UK: Cambridge University Press.

Stoel-Gammon, C., & Dunn, C. (1985). *Normal and disordered phonology in children.* Austin, TX: Pro-Ed.

Velten, H. V. (1971). The growth of phonemic and lexical patterns in the infant. Reprinted in A. Bar-Adon & W. Leopold (Eds.), *Readings in child language.* Englewood Cliffs, NJ: Prentice-Hall. (Originally published in 1941 in *Language, 19,* 440–444.)

Vihman, M. M. (1996). *Phonological development: The origins of language in the child.* Oxford: Basil Blackwell, Ltd.

Vihman, M., Macken, M. A., Miller, R., Simmons, H., & Miller, J. (1985). From babbling to speech: A re-assessment of the continuity issue. *Language, 61,* 397–445.

Vihman, M., & Miller, R. (1988). Words and babble at the threshold of language acquisition. In M. D. Smith and J. L. Locke (Eds.), *The emergent lexicon: The child's development of a linguistic vocabulary.* New York: Academic Press.

Waterson, N. (1971). Child phonology: A prosodic view. *Journal of Linguistics, 7,* 179–221.

Waterson, N. (1978). Growth of complexity in phonological development. In N. Waterson & C. E. Snow (Eds.), *The development of communication.* New York: Wiley.

Werker, J. F., & Pegg, J. E. (1992). Infant speech perception and phonological acquisition. In Ferguson, C., Menn, L., and Stoel-Gammon, C. (Eds.), *Phonological development: Models, research, implications.* Parkton, MD: York Press.

References

Atkinson, K. B., MacWhinney, B., & Stoel, C. (1970). An experiment in the recognition of babbling. *Papers and Reports in Child Language Development, 1,* 71–76.

Atkinson-King, K. (1973). Children's acquisition of phonological stress contrasts. *UCLA Working Papers in Phonetics, 25.*

Barton, D. P. (1980). Phonemic perception in children. In G. Yeni-Komshian, J. F. Kavanagh, & C. A. Ferguson (Eds.), *Child phonology: Vol. 2. Perception.* New York: Academic Press.

Bernstein Ratner, N. (1984a). Patterns of vowel modification in mother–child speech. *Journal of Child Language, 11,* 557–578.

Bernstein Ratner, N. (1984b). Cues to post-vocalic voicing in mother–child speech. *Journal of Phonetics, 12,* 285–289.

Best, C. T., McRoberts, G. W., & Sithole, N. M. (1988). Examination of the perceptual reorganization for speech contrasts: Zulu click discrimination. *Journal of Experimental Psychology: Perception and Performance, 14,* 245–360.

Boysson-Bardies, B. de, Sagart, L., & Durand, C. (1984). Discernible differences in the babbling of infants according to target language. *Journal of Child Language, 11,* 1–15.

Boysson-Bardies, B. de, & Vihman, M. M. (1991). Adaptation to language: Evidence from babbling and first words in four languages. *Language, 67,* 297–319.

Braine, M. D. S. (1974). On what might constitute a learnable phonology. *Language, 50,* 270–299.

Branigan, G. (1979). *Sequences of words as structured units.* Unpublished doctoral dissertation, Boston University School of Education.

Butler Platt, C., & MacWhinney, B. (1983). Solving a problem vs. remembering a solution: Error assimilation as a strategy in language acquisition. *Journal of Child Language, 10,* 41–75.

DeCasper, A. J., & Fifer, W. P. (1980). Of human bonding: Newborns prefer their mothers' voices. *Science, 208,* 1174–1176.

Deser, T. (1990). *Dialect transmission and variation: An acoustic analysis of vowels in six urban Detroit families.* Bloomington, IN: Indiana Linguistics Club Publications.

Dodd, B. J. (1972). Effects of social and vocal stimulation on infant babbling. *Developmental Psychology, 7,* 80–83.

Edwards, M. L., & Shriberg, L. D. (1983). *Phonology: Applications in communicative disorders* (pp. 123–199). San Diego, CA: College-Hill Press.

Eimas, P. D., Siqueland, E. R., Jusczyk, P., & Vigorito, J. (1971). Speech perception in infants. *Science, 171,* 303–306.

Ferguson, C. A., & Farwell, C. B. (1975). Words and sounds in early language acquisition. *Language, 51,* 439–491.

Ferguson, C. A., & Macken, M. A. (1980). Phonological development in children's play and cognition. In K. E. Nelson (Ed.), *Children's language* (Vol. 4). New York: Gardner Press.

Ferguson, C. A., Menn, L., & Stoel-Gammon, C. (Eds.). (1992). *Phonological development: Models, research, implications.* Parkton, MD: York Press.

Gerken, L., & McIntosh, B. (1993). The interplay of function morphemes and prosody in early language. *Developmental Psychology, 29,* 448–457.

Grunwell, P. (1987). *Clinical phonology* (2nd ed.). Baltimore: Williams and Wilkins.

Halliday, M. A. K. (1975). *Learning how to mean: Explorations in the development of language.* London: Edward Arnold.

Ingram, D. (1989). *Phonological disabilities in children.* (2nd ed.). London: Cole and Whurr.

Jaeger, J. J. (1980). *Categorization in phonology: An experimental approach.* Unpublished doctoral dissertation. Berkeley, CA: University of California.

Jakobson, R. (1968). *Child language, aphasia, and phonological universals.* (A. Keiler, Trans.). The Hague: Mouton (first published 1941).

Jesperson, O. (1925). *Language.* New York: Holt, Rinehart & Winston.

Jusczyk, P. W. (1992). Developing phonological categories for the speech signal. In Ferguson, C. A., Menn, L., & Stoel-Gammon, C. (Eds.). *Phonological development: Models, research, implications.* Parkton, MD: York Press.

Kuhl, P. K. (1992). Speech prototypes: Studies on the nature, function, ontogeny and phylogeny of the "centers" of speech categories. In Y. Tohkura, E. Vatikiotis-Bateson, & Y. Sagiska (Eds.) *Speech Perception, production and linguistic structure.* Tokyo: Ohmsha.

Krohn, R., Steinberg, D., & Kobayashi, L. (1972). The psychological validity of Chomsky and Halle's vowel shift rule. *20th International Congress of Psychology,* Tokyo (Abstract Guide, paragraph 1905).

Leonard, L. B. (1992). Models of phonological development and children with phonological disorders. In Ferguson, C. A., Menn, L., & Stoel-Gammon, C. (Eds.). *Phonological development: Models, research, implications.* Parkton, MD: York Press.

Leopold, W. (1970). *Speech development of a bilingual child, 1–4.* New York: AMS Press.

Lieberman, P., Crelin, E. S., & Klatt, D. H. (1972). Phonetic ability and related anatomy of the newborn, adult human, Neanderthal man, and the chimpanzee. *American Anthropologist, 74,* 287–307.

Lindblom, B. (1992). Phonological units as adaptive emergents of lexical development. In Ferguson, C. A., Menn, L., & Stoel-Gammon, C. (Eds.). *Phonological development: Models, research, implications.* Parkton, MD: York Press.

Locke, J. L. (1983). *Phonological acquisition and change.* New York: Academic Press.

Macken, M. A. (1979). Developmental reorganization of phonology: A hierarchy of basic units of acquisition. *Lingua, 49,* 11–49.

Macken, M. A. (1980). The child's lexical representation: The "puzzle-puddle-pickle" evidence. *Journal of Linguistics, 16,* 1–19.

Macken, M. A., & Barton, D. (1980). The acquisition of voicing contrast in English: A study of voice onset time in word-initial stop consonant. *Journal of Child Language, 7,* 41–75.

Macken, M. A., & Ferguson, C. A. (1983). Cognitive aspects of phonological development: model, evidence, and issues. In K. E. Nelson (Ed.), *Children's Language* (Vol. 4). Hillsdale, NJ: Lawrence Erlbaum Associates, Inc.

Malsheen, B. (1980). Two hypotheses for phonetic clarification in the speech of mothers to children. In G. Yeni-Komshian, J. F. Kavanagh, & C. A. Ferguson (Eds.), *Child phonology: Vol. 2. Perception.* New York: Academic Press.

McCawley, J. D. (1977). Acquisition models as models of acquisition. In R. Fasold & R. Shuy (Eds.), *Studies in language variation* (pp. 51–64). Washington, DC: Georgetown University Press.

Mehler, J., Jusczyk, P. W., Lambertz, G., Halsted, N., Bertoncini, J., & Amiel-Tisson, C. (1988). A precursor of language acquisition in young infants. *Cognition, 29,* 143–178.

Menn, L. (1971). Phonotactic rules in beginning speech. *Lingua, 26,* 225–241.

Menn, L. (1976). *Pattern, control, and contrast in beginning speech: A case study in the acquisition of word form and function.* Unpublished doctoral dissertation, University of Illinois.

Menn, L., & Matthei, E. (1992). The "two-lexicon" account of child phonology: Look back, looking ahead. In Ferguson, C. A., Menn, L., & Stoel-Gammon, C. (Eds.), *Phonological development: Models, research, implications.* Parkton, MD: York Press.

Moskowitz, A. I. (1970). The two-year-old stage in the acquisition of English phonology. *Language, 46,* 426–441.

Moskowitz, B. A. (1980). Idioms in phonology acquisition and phonological change. *Journal of Phonetics, 8,* 69–83.

Mowrer, O. H. (1954). The psychologist looks at language. *American Psychologist, 9,* 660–694.

Myerson, R. (1975). *A developmental study of children's knowledge of complex derived words of English.* Unpublished doctoral dissertation, Harvard Graduate School of Education.

Nakazima, S. A. (1962). A comparative study of the speech developments of Japanese and American English in childhood (1): A comparison of the developments of voices at the prelinguistic period. *Studia Phonologica, 2,* 27–46.

Nelson, K. (1973). Structure and strategy in learning to talk. *Monographs of the Society for Research in Child Development, 38.*

Oller, D. K. (1980). The emergence of the sounds of speech in infancy. In G. Yeni-Komshian, J. F. Kavanagh, & C. A. Ferguson (Eds.), *Child phonology: (Vol. 1). Production.* New York: Academic Press.

Oller, D. K., & Eilers, R. (1988). The role of audition in babbling. *Child Development, 59,* 441–449.

Olmsted, D. L. (1971). *Out of the mouth of babes.* The Hague: Mouton.

Olney, R. L., & Scholnick, E. K. (1976). Adult judgment of age and linguistic differences in infant vocalization. *Journal of Child Language, 3,* 145–156.

Painter, C. (1984). *Into the mother tongue: A case study in early language development.* London: Frances Pinter.

Payne, A. (1976). *The acquisition of a phonological system of a second dialect.* Unpublished doctoral dissertation, University of Pennsylvania.

Peters, A. M. (1977). Language learning strategies. *Language, 53,* 560–573.

Peters, A., & Menn, L. (1993). False starts and filler syllables: Way to learn grammatical morphemes. *Language, 69,* 742–777.

Prather, E., Hedrick, D., and Kern, C. (1975). Articulation development in children aged two to four years. *Journal of Speech and Hearing Disorders, 40,* 179–191.

Priestly, T. M. S. (1977). One idiosyncratic strategy in the acquisition of phonology. *Journal of Child Language, 4,* 45–66.

Rheingold, H. L., Gerwitz, J. L., & Ross, H. W. (1959). Social conditioning of vocalizations in the infant. *Journal of Comparative and Physiological Psychology, 52,* 68–73.

Schwartz, R. G., & Leonard, L. B. (1982). Do children pick and choose? An examination of phonological selection and avoidance in early lexical acquisition. *Journal of Child Language, 9,* 319–336.

Smit, A. B. (1993). Phonological error distributions in the Iowa-Nebraska articulation norms project: Word-initial consonant clusters. *Journal of Speech and Hearing Research, 36,* 931–947.

Smit, A. B. Hand, L., Freilinger, F. F., Bernthal, J. E., & Bird, A. (1990). The Iowa articulation norms project and its Nebraska replication. *Journal of Speech and Hearing Disorders, 55,* 779–798.

Smith, N. V. (1973). *The acquisition of phonology: A case study.* Cambridge, UK: Cambridge University Press.

Stampe, D. (1969). The acquisition of phonemic representation. *Proceedings of the Fifth Regional Meeting of the Chicago Linguistic Society,* pp. 433–444.

Stark, R. E. (1980). Stages of speech development in the first year. In G. Yeni-Komshian, J. A. Kavanagh, & C. A. Ferguson (Eds.), *Child phonology* (Vol. 1). New York: Academic Press.

Stemberger, J. P. (1992). A connectionist view of child phonology: Phonological processing without phonological processes. In Ferguson, C. A., Menn, L., & Stoel-Gammon, C. (Eds.), *Phonological development: Models, research, implications.* Parkton, MD: York Press.

Stoel-Gammon, C. (1985). Phonetic inventories, 15–24 months: A longitudinal study. *Journal of Speech and Hearing Research, 28,* 505–512.

Stoel-Gammon, C., & Dunn, C. (1985). *Normal and disordered phonology in children.* Austin, TX: Pro-Ed.

Stoel-Gammon, C., & Otomo, K. (1986). Babbling development of hearing-impaired and normally hearing subjects. *Journal of Speech and Hearing Disorders, 51,* 33–41.

Templin, M. C. (1957). Certain language skills in children: Their development and interrelationships. Minneapolis: University of Minnesota Press.

Todd, G., & Palmer, B. (1968). Social reinforcement of infant babbling. *Child Development, 39,* 591–596.

Trehub, S. E. (1976). The discrimination of foreign speech contrasts by infants and children. *Child Development, 47,* 466–472.

Velleman, S. (1988). The role of linguistic perception in later phonological development. *Journal of Applied Psycholinguistics, 9,* 221–236.

Vihman, M. M. (1992). Early syllables and the construction of phonology. In Ferguson, C. A., Menn, L., & Stoel-Gammon, C. (Eds.), *Phonological development: Models, research, implications.* Parkton, MD: York Press.

Vihman, M. M., Macken, M. A., Miller, R., Simmons, H., and Miller, J. (1985). From babbling to speech: A re-assessment of the continuity issue. *Language, 61,* 397–445.

Wahler, R. G. (1969). Infant social development: Some experimental analyses of an infant-mother interaction during the first year of life. *Journal of Experimental Child Psychology, 7,* 101–113.

Waterson, N. (1971). Child phonology: A prosodic view. *Journal of Linguistics, 7,* 179–221.

Weir, R. (1962). *Language in the crib.* The Hague: Mouton.

Weisberg, P. (1963). Social and nonsocial conditioning of infant vocalization. *Child Development, 39,* 377–388.

Werker, J. F., & Tees, R. C. (1984). Cross-language speech perception: Evidence for perceptual reorganization during the first year of life. *Infant Behavior and Development, 7,* 49–64.

Wilbur, R., & Menn, L. (1975). *Towards a redefinition of psychological reality: The internal structure of the lexicon* (Occasional Papers in Linguistics). San Jose, CA: San Jose State College.

Winitz, H. (1969). *Articulatory acquisition and behavior.* New York: Appleton-Century-Crofts.

Chapter Four

Semantic Development: Learning the Meanings of Words

Barbara Alexander Pan, *Harvard Graduate School of Education,*
Jean Berko Gleason, *Boston University*

Introduction

Infants understand some of what is said to them long before they know any words at all. This earliest comprehension is at the emotional level: The exaggerated prosodic contours of their mothers' speech carry varied messages of comfort, happiness, prohibition, or anger (Fernald, 1992; Locke, 1993). Very young children understand the pragmatic intent of adults' utterances before they can understand the individual words. A toddler who begins to peel off his clothes on hearing his father say, "It's time for your bath now," may be responding to a variety of situational cues—it is a particular time of day, they are in a certain room, they are engaged in a familiar activity, or the parent may actually be pointing to the bathtub. Only very slowly do children come to understand and use words in adult fashion, to break them free of context and use them flexibly in a variety of situations. The acquisition of words, their meanings, and the links between them does not usually happen at once. During the course of this process, which is usually called **semantic development,** children's strategies for learning word meanings and relating them to one another change as their internal representation of language constantly grows and becomes reorganized.

In this chapter we will describe the relationship between words and their referents, and some of the theories that attempt to explain how children acquire and represent meaning. We will address what is known about early words and the ways in which contemporary researchers have attempted to interpret the data on children's early words and word meanings. We will also present research on later semantic development, which examines the ways that the semantic system is elaborated as words become related to one another in more complex semantic networks. Finally, we will describe children's growing awareness of words as physical entities independent of their meanings, and discuss the implications of such **metalinguistic development** for a variety of nonliteral language uses.

The Relations between Words and Their Referents

What does it mean to say that children acquire meaning? And what is it that adults share when they know the meaning of a word? First, it is important to note that the meaning of a word resides in the speakers of a common language, not in the world of objects. The word is a sign that signifies a **referent,** but the referent is not the meaning of the word. If, for example, you say to a child, "Look at the kitty," the referent, the actual cat, is not the meaning of *kitty*—if the cat ran away or were run over by a truck, the word would still have meaning because meaning is an act of cognition.

Let us assume that a child learns that the word *kitty* refers to her cat; in this case, the actual cat is the referent of the word *kitty.* But what is the relationship between the word and the cat? Cats can be called *kitty, cat, koshka, macska, katze,* or *chat,* depending on whether one is speaking English, Russian, Hungarian, German, or French. There is nothing intrinsic to cats that makes one or another name more appropriate or fitting—the relationship between the name and the thing is thus *arbitrary,* and it is by social convention in a particular language that speakers agree to call the animal by a particular word (Morris, 1946). This arbitrary relationship between the referent (the cat) and the sign for it (the word *cat*) is *symbolic.* Nonverbal signs can also share this symbolic nature; the red light that means stop, for instance, is purely symbolic because there is no obvious connection between the color red and the action of stopping. We could agree to have blue lights or even green lights mean *stop,* as long as we all agreed on the meaning of the light.

For a few words, the relation between word and referent is not arbitrary. If one says, for example, "The book fell with a *thud,*" the relationship between the word *thud* and the actual sound referred to is not arbitrary, since the word resembles the sound. As well, the name of the cuckoo bird is not arbitrary: it represents the sound that the bird actually makes. Although the study of semantic acquisition has concentrated on how children learn the meaning of symbols, we should not be surprised to learn that many of children's earliest words or protowords have a less-than-arbitrary relation to their referents; clocks are called *tick-tock,* and painful bumps become *owies.* Some of these words are in the baby-talk lexicon that adults use when attempting to communicate with babies, and others are the children's own creations.

It is probably easier for children to learn a word that is obviously related to its referent than one that is totally arbitrary and symbolic; and, as some research has shown, young children believe that the name and the referent have more than a casual connection. They think that one cannot change the name of something without changing its nature as well; for instance, if one decided to call a dog a *cow*, a child might assume that the animal would begin to moo (Vygotsky, 1962).

This belief in the essential appropriateness of names was a subject of argument among ancient philosophers as well. Plato, writing in the fourth century B.C., discussed the question of whether there is a natural relation between names and referents in his Cratylus dialogue. The Anomalists of Plato's day believed that the relation was inexplicable, but the Analogists believed that through careful etymology the essential nature of words could be revealed (Bloomfield, 1933).

Using English examples, we might show that a blackberry is so called because it is a berry that is black, and a bedroom is so named because it is a room containing a bed. The ancient Greek Analogists would also claim that if we only looked hard enough, we would find the natural connections behind *gooseberry* and *mushroom* as well. This altogether human desire to produce order can be seen in many **folk etymologies** today, and explains why college students as well as young children, when asked why Friday is called *Friday*, may respond, "Because it is the day you eat fried fish," or why they may hold that a handkerchief is so named "Because you hold it in your hand and go *kerchoo*" (Berko, 1958).

Mental Images

Although meaning is a mental event, we still have to specify what its exact nature is. One possibility is that meaning is a mental picture. As we have seen earlier (see Chapter 1), incoming language is processed in the part of the brain known as Wernicke's area, which is near the auditory association areas of the brain. The belief that the sound of a word evokes a mental picture of its referent and that the image is the meaning of the word has a long history (see Tichener, 1909). However, even though it is true that many people are able to visualize and can imagine quite vivid pictures, not everyone does so.

There are many other reasons that mental images cannot be the same as meaning (Brown, 1968). Many words, such as *happy* or *jealousy*, do not have picturable referents, and still we know their meanings. In addition, even if one has an image for a word, it is liable to be quite particularistic—*dog*, for instance, might evoke a picture of a black poodle you know. Yet anyone who knows the meaning of *dog* can recognize many hundreds of real dogs of all sizes and shapes, so the mental image would have to be a very complicated composite if it had to account for all instances. Clearly, this is not the case. Finally, images tend to be quite idiosyncratic; speakers who share meaning may hold very different internal images. One speaker's mental house may look like a mansion, whereas another's may be a simple cottage, yet both speakers recognize new instances of houses when they encounter them.

Concepts

One of the child's primary tasks in semantic development is to acquire categorical concepts (e.g., to learn that the word *dog* refers to a whole class of animals). Theorists differ as to how they characterize the nature of children's categorical concept acquisition. One view is that children acquire categories defined by semantic features, a second is that they acquire probabilistic concepts, and yet another is that they acquire prototypes.

The **semantic feature** view is that children learn a set of distinguishing features for each categorical concept. For instance, children learn that the word *dog* refers to a category of animals that are alive and warm-blooded, have four legs, bark, and are covered with hair. According to Eve Clark (1974), when a child learns a new word, it is in the context of a specific situation. The word *dog* may at first be understood to apply only to the child's own dog, and only later comes the understanding that other creatures may also be called "dog" as long as they share the small set of critical features that uniquely define the category. Overextensions occur when the child infers category membership from a partial match of features. A toddler may, in this way, call a moose "doggie" because both animals have hair and four legs. According to feature theory, the child in this case does not yet know that antlers disqualify an animal from membership in the dog category.

Some researchers, notably Smith and Medin (1981), have pointed out that even if children are acquiring their concepts as categories, there are great differences in the nature of the concepts themselves. For instance, there are **classical concepts**, like "bachelor"; every instance of this concept must have the qualities of being male, adult, and unmarried. One cannot meet, for instance, a married bachelor. The concept "triangle" is another example of a classical concept; all triangles must have three angles, or they are simply not triangles.

In contrast to classical concepts, there are also **probabilistic concepts**, like "bird." Most birds have feathers and beaks, fly, chirp, etc., but not all do. For instance, a kiwi is a nonflying bird. Concepts that involve people are often probabilistic: "doctor," for example. All instances (doctors) share some characteristics, like some medical training, but other characteristics, like "has high self-esteem," are typical of only some doctors (Smith & Medin, 1981).

Some examples of probabilistic concepts have more of the qualities of the concept than others. For example, a robin has more typical "bird" characteristics than does a penguin—therefore, people see robins as better examples of birds, and they also can classify them faster when asked if a robin is a bird. These typical examples of the category, or **prototypes,** are more accessible in memory in adult subjects (Rosch, 1973). According to prototype theory (see Figure 4.1), children acquire these core concepts when they acquire meaning and only later come to recognize members of that category that are distant from the prototypes. Andrick and Tager-Flusberg (1986)

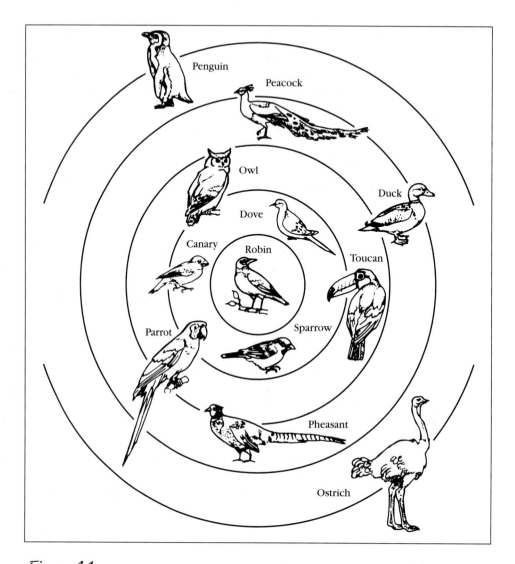

Figure 4.1

Some birds are more prototypical than others (From *Words in the Mind* [p. 54] by J. Aitchison, 1987. London: Basil Blackwell. Adapted by permission.)

found that **focal colors**—the bluest blues and the reddest red—were most easily named by children.

We have come a long way from the notion that meaning might be a little picture in one's brain. Next we consider behavioral and developmental theories of how children acquire words and their meanings.

Theoretical Perspectives on Semantic Development

Behavioral Theory

One of the simplest explanations of how children <u>learn the meanings</u> of their first words is that they do so <u>through association</u>. This behavioral model is very similar to the classical conditioning model proposed by learning theorists for any kind of associative learning (see Chapter 7 for further discussion of this theory). In learning through association, there is first an unconditioned stimulus that produces a response. In Pavlov's famous experiments, dogs were first presented with meat powder (the unconditioned stimulus), which caused the quite natural response of salivating. Later, a bell was rung at the same time that the powder was presented. Eventually, the dogs salivated when the bell rang, even when there was no meat powder present. The dogs responded to the sound of the bell, at least in part, as they had responded to the meat powder. They had become conditioned to the bell, which had thus become the conditioned stimulus.

How might this model be extended to cover the acquisition of meaning? If we assume that the infant already has some responses to objects in the world, then through a similar process of association the names of the objects can be learned. For example, the baby is familiar with the family cat and has certain expectations whenever it appears. If the parent points and says "kitty," eventually the infant will react to the word alone (at least in part), as if the cat were there—looking around for it or feeling pleased and ready for play. The cat, in this model, is the unconditioned stimulus that gives rise to certain predispositions or responses in the child. Eventually, the word *kitty* becomes the conditioned stimulus that evokes much the same set of responses.

It is important to remember that the conditioned response is similar to, but not really the same as, the original response to the unconditioned stimulus (Lashley, 1954). Pavlov's dogs may have salivated at the sound of the bell as they had salivated at the sight of the meat powder, but they did not try to eat the bell. The infant may respond somewhat to the word *kitty* as if it were the actual cat, but not to the extent of patting the empty air. For learning to have taken place, it suffices that the word *kitty* and the actual cat have been associated so that they evoke at least some of the same responses. Association theory may explain the earliest and simplest kinds of linking between words and objects. Many of children's early words, such as *bottle* and *blanket,* <u>have concrete referents and could be learned through association</u>. The acquisition of more abstract early words, such as *more,* requires a more complex explanation.

Developmental Theories

In contrast to the behavioral model, developmental theories consider semantic development within the wider context of the child's general cognitive and linguistic skills. Such theories attempt to explain how the child may acquire first words, why the scope of reference to which children's early words are applied may not match that of adults, and how children's semantic systems become more adultlike over time. It is clear that young children <u>first acquire meaning in a very context-bound way</u>, as a part of their real-world expectations. As research on prelinguistic development has shown, by the time children begin to understand language and to talk, their cognitive development has made significant strides. Researchers like John Macnamara (1972) have pointed out that very young children map language onto a set of observations about the world that they have already made. They do not learn about taking baths because their parents say, "It's bath time"; rather, they already know that their daily routine contains such an item, and at some point they realize that the parent's phrase refers to that familiar activity. Clark (1993) theorizes that before they start learning language, all children have developed a set of **ontological categories** (concepts about how the world is organized). These ontological categories include objects, actions, events, relations, states, and properties. These are the basic categories in all languages that speakers refer to when they use language.

Even before we can talk about the nature of children's conceptual categories, however, we need to appreciate the magnitude of the task facing an infant poised on the threshold of verbal communication. What must a nine-month-old understand about verbal communication in order to begin mapping words she hears to referents? Let us say, for instance, that an infant is in her home, and the family dog Rufus is lying nearby on a rug with a bone. The baby hears her mother say words such as *Rufus, dog, bone* and *look*. In the child's early experience, a word may apply only to the single referent she hears mentioned in discourse; for instance, *dog* might mean only her own family's dog. Most theorists and researchers would agree, however, that young children must come to understand that a single label can be applied to more than one specific case (that is, *dog* refers not only to their own Rufus, but to many different dogs, seen in the park, pictured in books and on dog food boxes, etc.). Without this insight, infants cannot begin to understand the nature of reference, or to communicate about objects, actions, and properties (Clark, 1993). However, this understanding is only one step in cracking the mapping puzzle. Not only does the label *dog* refer to many different dogs, but a particular dog may be labeled in many different ways (*Rufus, dog, retriever, pet, puppy*). Moreover, when a child hears a new word, the word could refer to an action, a property, or even a part of an object.

Constraints

To explain how young children may avoid this mapping nightmare, theorists have suggested **principles** or **constraints** that children may use as working hypotheses about the meanings of new words.

- *Words refer to objects.* One basic hypothesis young children may have is that when they hear a new word, it probably refers to an object, that is, to a person, place, or thing (Golinkoff, Mervis, & Hirsh-Pasek, 1994). This working hypothesis could sometimes lead to inaccurate mappings (when, for example, the parent points at a bird and says "Look!", rather than "Birdie!"). It would probably more often result in correct mappings, however, given that adults talking to young children produce more nouns than verbs (Goldfield, 1993).

- *Words refer to whole objects.* A second, related, hypothesis children may have is that when they hear a new label it refers to a *whole object,* rather than to its parts (Macnamara, 1982; Markman & Wachtel, 1988). This principle would predispose the child to eliminate the family dog's floppy ears or his appealing expression as likely referents for the new label *bone.* Because young children seem to rely heavily on shape to identify whole objects, this hypothesis has also been referred to as a **shape bias** (Landau, Smith, & Jones, 1988).

- *New words refer to categories that do not already have a name.* Golinkoff and her colleagues (1994) suggest that on hearing a new label, children will try to map the label to an as-yet-unlabeled object in the environment (**novel name-nameless category principle**). Thus, the child might assume that the new label *bone* referred to either the bone or the rug the dog is lying on (if the child did not yet know either of these words). As the child acquires more and more labels, the number of unlabeled referents in any given setting decreases, and the mapping task becomes easier.

- *No two words have exactly the same meaning.* Clark (1987) proposes a slightly different child principle, that is, that words contrast in meaning. According to this **principle of contrast,** the child would not completely eliminate Rufus as a possible referent for the new label *bone,* but would assume that the meaning of the word *bone* did not overlap perfectly with the meaning of the word *Rufus.*

- *Each object can have only one name.* Markman and her colleagues (Markman, 1987; Markman & Wachtel, 1988) propose a more stringent constraint than the one proposed by Clark, that is, that children assume an object can have only one name. According to this **principle of mutual exclusivity** there is no overlap between words. In our example, this would lead the child to eliminate Rufus as a possible referent for *bone,* because Rufus already has a name.

Although the proposed constraints or principles differ in their particulars, each suggests that learning the meaning of new words involves some process of comparing new to old semantic knowledge and incorporating the new mapping into a preexisting semantic system made up of other label-to-referent mappings. Ultimately, these complex relations will become **semantic networks,** as we shall see in later sections of this chapter.

As children grow older, they are able to use both linguistic and world knowledge to supplement or override their semantic predispositions. For example, Au and Glusman (1990) found that children who heard the novel material term *rattan* contrasted with other material terms ("It's not paper, and it's not cloth; it's rattan.") were more likely to learn the new material name than were children who simply heard rattan labeled. Hall (1994a) showed that three-year-olds assumed that *zav* was a proper name in a sentence such as "This dog is zav," but interpreted it as an adjective in the sentence, "This caterpillar is zav." Even three-year-olds knew that it was likely that a dog had a proper name, but that a caterpillar did not, and were able to use this world knowledge to interpret the new word. Regardless of what hypotheses children adopt, they will occasionally make incorrect initial mappings. As we will see later, children rely on input and feedback from mature speakers to test and revise their label-to-referent mappings.

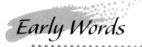

Early Words

Early in their second year, most children have begun to produce some words themselves. They begin with words related to what is intellectually and socially most meaningful to them (Anglin, 1995), such as names for important people and objects in their lives. Thus *mommy, daddy, doggie,* and *blankey* are common early words, and *tree, vase,* and *policeman* are not. Subsequent patterns of word meaning and use reflect development not only within children's semantic systems, but also in other areas such as their cognition and memory, in addition to widened experience.

The Study of Vocabulary

Examination of children's vocabulary is probably the oldest approach to the study of language acquisition. Beginning word use signals that children have a new tool that will enable them to learn about and participate more fully in their societies. Furthermore, word use is thought to provide tangible indicators of the makeup and workings of children's minds. The first studies—some as early as the eighteenth century (e.g., Tiedemann, 1787)—were almost invariably based on observations of the authors' own children and were kept in the form of diaries. During the nineteenth century and the first half of the twentieth century, many psychologists kept diary records of their children's development. This remains a valuable way to trace the development of language in individual children. One of the most famous diary studies was conducted by Werner Leopold (1970), whose four-volume work traced the development of both English and German in his daughter Hildegarde:

> Hildegarde was from birth exposed to two languages, English and German, simultaneously, and built her own early speech from selected vocabulary items from both

languages.... In examining Hildegarde's vocabulary it is necessary to keep in mind that meanings are necessarily hazy and vague at first.... (Leopold, 1948, p. 174)

Diaries can be a valuable adjunct to other research on children's language. By themselves, however, they can be misleading, since the temptation to write what is unusual or interesting, rather than what is daily and ordinary, is hard to resist. More recently, a number of researchers have found ways to augment and improve diary studies, by giving parents who are participating in a study checklists of the words that their children are likely to acquire during their first years (Dale, Bates, Reznick, & Morisset, 1989). The checklists help parents organize their observations and remind them of the more ordinary, but important, things their children understand and say that they might otherwise overlook.

What Are Early Words Like?

By the time children begin to acquire a vocabulary, they have already been exposed to a great deal of language and have had a wide range of individual experiences. It is interesting, therefore, that children's initial productive or expressive vocabularies have been found to be quite similar, despite differences in upbringing and environment.

The words children acquire in their early productive vocabularies are influenced by many factors. One of these factors is phonological composition. Researchers have analyzed the phonology of children's first fifty words (Ferguson & Farwell, 1975; Stoel-Gammon & Cooper, 1984), studied children's imitations of words (Leonard, Schwartz, Folger, Newhoff, & Wilcox, 1979), and tried to teach new words to one-year-olds (Leonard, Schwartz, Morris, & Chapman, 1981; Schwartz & Leonard, 1982). The results of these studies show that words that are easier for children to pronounce are more likely to be included in their early productive vocabularies, and that favored sound patterns may vary greatly across children. Moreover, phonological composition continues to play a role in vocabulary through the early school years. Unlike adults, children aged five to seven tend to use few words that sound very similar to one another (Charles-Luce & Luce, 1990).

From the beginning, children's vocabularies appear to include words from a variety of grammatical classes; their first fifty words represent all of the major grammatical classes found in adult language (see Table 4.1).

Nonetheless, common nouns predominate in young children's early speech. Nearly 40 percent of the average child's first fifty words are common nouns, while verbs, adjectives, and function words each account for less than 10 percent (Bates, Marchman, Thal, Fenson, Dale, Reznick, Reilly, & Hartung, 1994). The tendency to favor nouns continues until children have amassed between one and two hundred words, by which time nouns account for 55 percent of the average child's vocabulary. Thereafter, verbs and adjectives, and later, function words begin to be added more rapidly, so that by the time children's productive vocabularies exceed 600 words,

Table 4.1	Children's Earliest Words: Examples from the Vocabularies of Children Younger than 20 Months.

Sound effects
  baa baa, meow, moo, ouch, uh-oh, woof, yum-yum
Food and drink
  apple, banana, cookie, cheese, cracker, juice, milk, water
Animals
  bear, bird, bunny, dog, cat, cow, duck, fish, kitty, horse, pig, puppy
Body parts and clothing
  diaper, ear, eye, foot, hair, hand, hat, mouth, nose, toe, tooth, shoe
House and outdoors
  blanket, chair, cup, door, flower, keys, outside, spoon, tree, tv
People
  baby, daddy, gramma, grampa, mommy, [child's own name]
Toys and vehicles
  ball, balloon, bike, boat, book, bubbles, plane, truck, toy
Actions
  down, eat, go, sit, up
Games and routines
  bath, bye, hi, night-night, no, peekaboo, please, shhh, thank you, yes
Adjectives and descriptives
  allgone, cold, dirty, hot

about 40 percent are nouns, 25 percent verbs and adjectives, and about 15 percent function words. Of course, these proportions vary from child to child. The nature of individual differences will be discussed in Chapter 8.

Why should nouns initially be acquired more rapidly than other types of words? Several possible explanations have been suggested. One hypothesis holds that children's vocabularies reflect the input directed to them; studies have shown that in adult speech to children, labels for different kinds of objects are more numerous than labels for actions, properties, or relations (Goldfield, 1993). An alternative explanation is that nouns are favored over verbs in acquisition because verbs are more linguistically complex. In addition, the concepts referred to by nouns are clearer, more concrete, and more readily identifiable than those of verbs (Gentner, 1983, 1988). Nouns tend to refer to the same concepts in different languages, but the particular aspects of meaning covered by verbs are not identical in different languages. Learning a verb's meaning requires a child to find out which of the possible aspects are included and which are not. The linguistic and conceptual complexity of verbs may be one reason

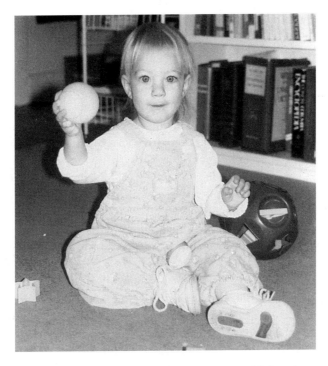

Words like "ball" that are easy to pronounce are likely to be in children's early vocabularies.

that children initially rely on general-purpose verbs such as *do, go, make,* and *get* (Clark, 1993). Comprehension and production of decontextualized verbs (those that do not refer to the here and now) appear to be particularly late to emerge (Smith & Sachs, 1990).

Although children's early vocabularies are quite varied, Bloom and Lahey (1978) found that children whose vocabularies are at the fifty-word level may actually use only eight or ten of those words very frequently and in a variety of contexts. Bloom and Lahey refer to this group of words as the **core group.** Children's vocabularies also include another group of less-favored words, somewhat greater in number, that are used at least once every day or two. The remaining vocabulary words are used rarely, perhaps as infrequently as once in a few months. Rescorla (1980) found in a longitudinal study that by the time her subjects had produced 445 words, 5 percent of those words had not been used for two months.

Unconventional Word/Meaning Mappings

An **overextension** is said to occur when a child uses a word in a context or manner that is inconsistent with, but in some way related to, the adult meaning of the word, as when a dog is called "kitty" or a cotton ball "snow," or when a visitor is greeted with a hearty "bye-bye!" Thus, the term *overextension* derives from the fact that the child is extending the term beyond the adult word concept. An **underextension** is said to occur when a child uses a particular word for only a limited subset of the contexts allowed by the adult concept. A child who saw many breeds of dogs but referred only to basset hounds, dachshunds, and corgis as "doggie" would appear to be extending the term to a reduced set of referents. Clark (1987), Mervis and Mervis (1988), and others have pointed out that children's categories may not initially match those of adults; they may use "duck" for birds that swim, "bird" for those that fly, and "chicken" for those that don't fly (Clark, 1987). Both overextensions and underextensions are common in one- and two-year-old children's speech, accounting for up to one-third of their production vocabulary (Clark, 1993). Beyond age two-and-a-half, however, such unconventional mappings become less noticeable.

What do children's extensions of words tell us? At best, they reveal how children categorize the world and what aspects of their experiences they find relevant to certain words. We might be able to detect ways in which children integrate their experiences differently than adults do. At the same time, some caution must also be exercised. As some researchers (e.g., Hoek, Ingram, & Gibson, 1986) have noted, the extent to which the child's spoken word should be considered an accurate representation of her inner structuring of the world remains unclear.

Although some overextensions occur because children's underlying word concepts differ from those of adults, other plausible explanations exist. As noted earlier, not all categories have clear-cut boundaries. Carabine (1991) found that most of the inappropriate labeling by two- and three-year-old children he studied consisted of labels applied to objects that were not uniformly categorized by adults either. In addition, some of children's overextensions may reflect retrieval problems, such that an older, better-known label (e.g., "dog") may be inappropriately used in place of a more recently acquired, but more appropriate one such as "moose" (Hoek, Ingram, & Gibson, 1986). At other times, children may not yet have acquired the proper label, even though their concepts match those of adults. They may then opt to use words as analogies or as semantic stand-ins for the words they do not know.

Nelson and her colleagues (Nelson, Benedict, Gruendel, & Rescorla, 1977) have suggested that young children are actively engaged in the "classification and cross-classification of features of . . . objects and events" and use their single words analogically to comment on similarities they have noticed. Thus, the child who points to a Saint Bernard and says "cow" is thought to mean only that the dog is *like* a cow. Hudson and Nelson (1984) have shown that two-year-olds who correctly label an object in a naming task may misname or substitute another label in pretend play. Additional evidence that children are using analogy comes from the fact that they are seldom observed to use words in this fashion after they acquire syntax and can explain what they mean.

In other situations, children seem to overextend words as a humorous gesture. When our two-year-old friend Matthew was shown a flying helicopter by his father, who pointed and said "helicopter," Matthew grinned, giggled, and said "airplane." Matthew's demeanor and the fact that he had used the word *helicopter* previously suggest that he was using his knowledge of words to make a joke. Determining what a child's early words mean requires attention to the contexts in which they are spoken and understood, as well as information about how the child has referred to the concepts or used the words before. Recent research thus shows that children's overextensions are not simply a reflection of incomplete categorization skills. Overextensions may be retrieval errors, semantic stand-ins, analogies, or even jokes.

Invented Words

In an early study, Berko (1958) found that preschoolers and first-graders were often able to invent words to refer to meanings that were specified by an experimenter. In this structured situation, children and adults were asked questions like "What would you call a man who 'zibs' for a living?" Although children only rarely employed the typical adult strategy of creating **derived words** by adding suffixes (a *zibber* zibs for a living), they were frequently able to create words by using alternative techniques (e.g., making **compound words** like *zib-man*).

Children also often invent or coin words spontaneously in their own speech. Sometimes invented words are used interchangeably with conventional words, as, for example, when a child uses *bee-house* and *bee-hive* in the same sentence (Becker, 1994). At other times, children may invent new words to fill gaps in their vocabularies (Clark, 1982). Clark found that these gaps occurred when the child had forgotten or did not know the usual word. Inventions such as *pourer* for *cup* and *plant-man* for *gardener* were common. Preschoolers frequently created needed verbs from nouns they knew, as when one child said, while putting crackers in her soup, "I'm crackering my soup" (Clark, 1981, p. 304).

Clark found that children's lexical innovations follow fairly regular principles. These are:

- **Simplicity.** Simplicity is reflected in children's use of a conventional word in an unconventional, but totally obvious, role (for example, *to pillow,* meaning "to throw a pillow at"; Clark, 1993, p. 120).

- **Semantic transparency.** Semantic transparency is evident in innovations such as *plant-man* for *gardner;* the meaning of the invented word is more apparent and more easily remembered than the conventional one.

- **Productivity.** Productivity is shown in children's use of forms that are frequently used by adults as the basis of new words. Many English words meaning "people who do something," for instance, end in *-er (teacher, player)*. Thus, children create agentival nouns such as *cooker,* and *bicycler.*

Differences between Comprehension and Production

According to Nelson and her colleagues (1977), comprehension of a word requires that a child, on hearing the word, anticipate or do something. Production of a word requires on its most basic level that the child speak the word at an appropriate time and place.

It was once believed that a child's productive or expressive vocabulary did not differ from his receptive or comprehension vocabulary except in size. Productive vocabularies do indeed typically lag behind receptive vocabularies; the children studied by Benedict (1979) comprehended their first fifty words at about thirteen months of age, but had not produced fifty words until about nineteen months. The differences between receptive and expressive vocabularies, however, involve not only rate of acquisition, but strategies as well. Researchers including Gruendel (cited in Nelson, Benedict, Gruendel, & Rescorla, 1977), Huttenlocher (1974), Rescorla (1981), and Thompson and Chapman (1977) have observed numerous examples of accurate word comprehension with a concurrent lack of differentiation in the productive vocabulary. One of Rescorla's subjects, Rachel, was able to identify a motorcycle, bike, truck, plane, and helicopter; yet at the same time she referred to them all as "car"!

For many years, researchers interested in investigating young children's vocabulary comprehension relied on tasks requiring the child to select or point to an object or picture labeled by the researcher. This methodology was less than ideal for at least two reasons. First, referents for some words, such as action verbs, are often difficult to depict. Second, infants and young children often do not reliably touch or point to the referent requested, even when their looking behaviors suggest they recognize the referent being labeled. Recently, researchers have begun using a new method, called the **preferential looking paradigm,** to test infants' and toddlers' vocabulary comprehension (Golinkoff, Hirsh-Pasek, Cauley, & Gordon, 1987). In this paradigm, the infant is seated on his blindfolded mother's lap facing two video monitors (see Chapter 5). Words or sentences are played over a centrally located speaker. At the same time, brief segments of videotape are shown on the two monitors. The object or action sequence shown on one monitor matches the word or sentence the child hears, while that shown on the other screen does not. Because children prefer to gaze at video segments matching what they hear, they will look longer at the matching screen if they understand the word or sentence. Using this method, Naigles and Gelman (1995) have recently found that children who call *cow* "doggie" nonetheless look longer at the picture of a cow than the competing picture of a dog, thus supporting results reported earlier by Thompson and Chapman (1977) and by Rescorla (1981).

Clearly, then, the receptive and expressive systems do not overlap perfectly, and a clear understanding of the dimensions and features of each requires careful study.

Features of Adult Speech That Influence Children's Semantic Development

Even before children begin using words themselves, adults' labeling and gaze behaviors serve to focus children's attention on objects. Much of adult speech addressed to young children deals with the here and now (Cross, 1977; Phillips, 1973; Shatz & Gelman, 1973; Snow, 1972). When adults look at and label objects that are visible to children, children assume the label refers to the adult focus of attention, and make an initial object-label mapping (Baldwin, 1991). This dovetailing of adults' and children's predispositions may help explain how children as young as thirteen months learn to comprehend new words after only a few exposures (Woodward, Markman, & Fitzsimmons, 1994). Adults also give children many opportunities to practice producing object labels themselves by engaging them in naming games (Ninio & Bruner, 1978). In these interactions, the parent points to and names specific objects for the child and then helps the child say the name.

The labels adults provide for children are not always the ones they would use with adults or older children. Anglin (1977, 1978) showed that adults vary their object labeling according to the audience. When asked to label a set of pictures of objects for two-year-olds, adults used general names like *money* instead of *nickel,* and *dog* instead of *collie.* Anglin also gave the adults sets of words at different levels of generality and asked them to group them according to the way they thought two-year-olds would categorize them. The adults' picture labeling for the children had the same patterns as their ratings of two-year-olds' categorizations. Thus, it appears that adults have preconceived notions of the minds and activities of two-year-olds and use labels that reflect those notions.

Adults sometimes mislabel objects when speaking to very young children, teaching them in some cases to use labels that are incorrect by adult standards. Mervis and Mervis (1982) gave ten mothers and their thirteen-month-olds sets of toys to play with and recorded their speech. The mothers named almost all of the toys for their children, and were observed quite often to misname some of them according to how their children might have categorized them. For example, a toy leopard was commonly referred to as "kitty-cat," and a toy tow truck was referred to as "car." Why would parents mislabel objects for their children? According to Mervis and Mervis, children provide their parents with signals indicating how they might categorize objects. Although babies first treat all objects in the same ways (mouthing, touching, shaking, and banging them), eventually they begin treating them differentially. At this point a doll might be held and a toy car pushed on the floor. Children's differential treatment of objects indicates on a fundamental level how they are categorizing the objects. By labeling the objects for children according to the children's own categories, parents are probably showing how words are used. That is, objects that differ in minor ways but are of the same category share names.

The naming practices of mothers seem to be based on children's own ways of categorizing the world (Golinkoff, Shuff-Bailey, Olguin, & Ruan, 1995). The names chosen follow what Rosch et al. (1976) have called **basic level categories.** The first principle underlying such categories is that similarities within categories are emphasized, rather than similarities between categories. Thus, because leopards are more like cats than other objects, they are labeled "cats." The second principle defining the basic level is that it is the most general level at which objects are similar because of their forms, functions, component parts (Poulin-Dubois, 1995), or motions. Thus, although an owl bank and a Christmas ornament share neither name nor function for adults, because they are round objects that would most likely be treated similarly (i.e., rolled) by very young children, they were grouped with balls and identified as "ball" by the mothers studied by the Mervises.

Mothers of young children use different strategies when teaching their children basic level terms than when they teach either more general or more specific terms (Callanan, 1985; Hall, 1994b). For basic level words, mothers use **ostension;** they may point and say, "That's a tractor." When asked to teach superordinates, however, they employ a strategy of *inclusion,* mentioning both basic level terms and the superordinate term. For instance, they say things such as "A car and a bus and a train. All of them are kinds of *vehicles.*" When teaching terms such as *passenger,* which are more specific than basic level terms, mothers provide an explanation that includes a basic level term as well as the new word. For example, they may say, "The pig is a passenger because he's riding in a car" or "A passenger is a person when he is riding in a car."

Mothers' speech has also been shown to have an effect on the ways that children come to understand and use vocabulary relating to their own inner states (Beeghly, Bretherton, & Mervis, 1986; Tingley, Gleason, & Hooshyar, 1994). In a study conducted in Great Britain, Dunn, Bretherton, and Munn (1987) found that mothers talking with their young children routinely labeled a variety of the children's inner states, including quality of consciousness (e.g., "bored"), physiological states ("dizzy"), and emotional states ("happy"). By the age of two, the children used many of these inner-state words themselves, particularly those relating to sleep, distress, dislike, temperature, pain, and pleasure. An even more intriguing finding of this study was that mothers used more of these labels with daughters, and, by the age of two, girls themselves referred to feeling states significantly more frequently than boys did.

In addition to the special vocabulary directed to young children, adults and even older children (Shatz & Gelman, 1973) seem to tailor other aspects of their language to the child's ability level; some of the characteristics of input language may facilitate semantic development. Input language, especially when young children begin to understand and use words, is more clearly and slowly enunciated and is characterized by exaggerated intonation and clear pauses between utterances (Sachs, Brown, & Salerno, 1976). In addition, sentence elements are often uttered in an isolated fashion (Newport, 1975; Snow, 1972), and words that are being taught or focused on tend to be placed in sentence-final position with especially marked pitch and stress (Fernald

& Mazzie, 1991). Thus, speech directed to young children tends to be better formed and more intelligible than speech to other adults, which tends to be fraught with sloppily pronounced words, false starts, and ill-formed or incomplete sentences with unclear boundaries between words. This clearer, more precise, and simpler input language could assist children in separating words from the flow of speech and in perceiving correct pronunciation. Similarly, the consistent pronunciation could aid them in becoming familiar with new words and in picking out those words that map meanings they wish to express.

Adults communicate with young children in order to share information about social, emotional, and physical topics, but in so doing, they provide children with feedback about their own language. Some feedback is nonverbal, as for example, when a mother appears when her child calls "mama" from the crib, or brings the child a saltine when he asks for a "cracker." If the child really wanted a cookie instead of a cracker, he will have made a useful (if disappointing) discovery. Corrective feedback can also be in verbal form. For example, when a child labels a yo-yo "ball," the adult may provide the correct label, accompanied by a description of critical features (e.g., "That's a yo-yo. See? It goes up and down"). Chapman, Leonard, and Mervis (1986) found that these types of corrections were the most effective in correcting children's overextensions.

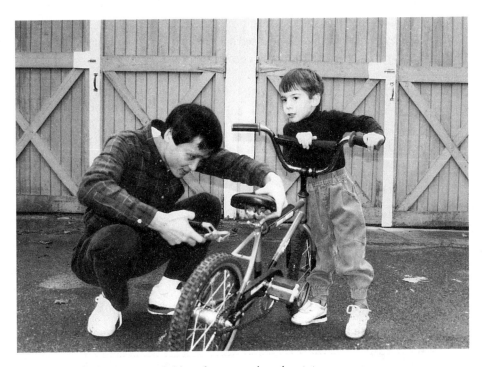

Much of adults' language to children focuses on shared activity.

Later Semantic Development

Complex Concepts

As we noted earlier, not all concepts are of comparable complexity; concrete object categories tend to be easier concepts to acquire than are action or affective categories, and superordinates are more difficult than are basic level categories. Other categories may be difficult to discriminate because they share many semantic features. **Kinship terms** exemplify this situation since many of them, such as *aunt* and *uncle,* share all but one feature.

Clark proposed a semantic feature hypothesis that predicted that terms whose meanings are defined by many features would be more difficult for children to master than terms that are semantically less complex. To test this hypothesis, Haviland and Clark (1974) asked children between the ages of three and eight to define English kinship terms. They asked questions like "What is an uncle?" or "What is a grandfather?" Terms that have only one relational component (e.g., *father:* a parent who is male) were expected to be less difficult than terms defined by many features (e.g., *aunt*). As expected, children learned the less complex kinship terms earlier, regardless of whether they had experience with the particular relationship. Haviland and Clark found that children's order of acquisition could be described in terms of adding component features, and that acquisition proceeded through four stages (see also earlier work by Danziger, 1957, and Piaget, 1928). At the earliest stage, one typical child (at three years, five months) has no component features:

Stage 1.

Q: "What's a cousin?"

A: "I have a cousin Daniel."

Q: "Are cousins big or little?"

A: "No."

Stage 2.

In the second stage, a child describes some features of the term but not relational ones, as in this example from a child of five years, ten months:

Q: "What's a father?"

A: "A father is somebody who goes to work every day except Saturday and Sunday and earns money."

Stage 3.

At the third stage, relational terms are used, but they are not yet reciprocal, as exemplified in this conversation with a child of six years, six months:

Q: "What's a mother?"

A: "It's a mommy. I have a mommy. It's somebody in your family."

Stage 4.

Finally, as with this seven-year-old, the child knows that the term is both relational and reciprocal:

Q: "What's a niece?"

A: "A niece is like a mother had a sister, and I'd be her niece."

Another type of complex concept that has received the attention of researchers is *deixis*. **Deictic terms** are pointers or contrasting relational terms that are used to indicate which of multiple objects is being referred to. The chief acquisitional challenge lies in the fact that the reference points for such terms depend upon who says them. Thus, for example, understanding the terms *I* and *you,* and *this* and *that,* requires that the speaker, rather than a fixed point, be assumed as the point of reference against which the meaning of the terms can be interpreted.

Some researchers have been interested in the acquisition of deictic terms for insights it might provide into the developmental relationship between cognition and language (deVilliers & deVilliers, 1974; Webb & Abrahamson, 1976). Comprehension of deictic terms would appear to require the type of multiple-perspective-taking ability that Piagetians maintain only becomes possible when children reach the stage of concrete operations, usually around seven years of age, However, deVilliers and deVilliers (1974) reported that three- and four-year-old preschoolers were able to use different points of view to employ deictic terms such as *here* and *there*. They also found that differences in perspective-taking demands made by different pairs of relative terms had acquisitional consequences. Their three-year-old subjects could comprehend terms that required them to assume the speaker's perspective; their four-year-old subjects could, in addition, correctly produce terms that required them to assume the listener's perspective. In addition, even though the meanings of terms that do not usually require a shift in perspective (e.g., *in front of* and *behind*) were acquired first, they became less well understood for a time when the children were beginning to take into account the effect of perspective on the meanings of other relational terms.

Clark and Sengul (1978), in another study of deictic terms, focused on the different interpretive strategies children employ along the path to full comprehension. Noting that both shifting reference perspective and the proximity of the referent to the speaker and listener combine in the meanings of deictic terms, they developed hypotheses about possible developmental paths. Their data indicated three stages in the acquisition of the deictic contrasts they studied: (1) a stage in which the terms are used with no deictic contrast (*there* is thought to mean *all done,* and *here* is used as a general referent indicator, or *here* and *there* are thought to be synonyms), (2) a stage in which children include some of the necessary contrasts (i.e., they understand the terms in some contexts only), and (3) a stage in which the requisite contrasts are encoded in the lexicon. The active role children play in their own semantic development was highlighted in this study. It was observed that there were differences among children in their initial implicit hypotheses about the words' meanings, as indicated by their response strategies. In choosing a toy that was "here" or "there," some children always chose the one that was near them, whereas others always chose the one that was near the speaker, regardless of the term that was used. These early strategies determined how they later interpreted the deictic terms.

Another example of how children acquire concept-label mappings for complex concepts is their acquisition of **color terms.** The conceptual knowledge required to learn the meanings of color terms includes being able, for analytic purposes, to isolate color from objects, differentiate among hues, and notice similarities among related shades. Linguistically, the child must know that color words refer to the dimension of color rather than, for instance, size (Bartlett, 1977). Color terms are somewhat unusual in that they (like number terms) may be recognized by children before the terms are connected to their referents. For example, when asked to group similar objects, two-year-olds who know no color words can use color as the basis for grouping (Soja, 1994). Likewise, well before they correctly and reliably answer the question "What color is this?", many children supply *some* color term. Once children begin to use color terms correctly, they generally do so in an order that some researchers say reflects a universal hierarchy (Berlin & Kay, 1969), but which others suggest may reflect parental patterns of use. Recent research (Gleason & Ely, 1996) has shown that the colors referred to by parents overlap with the basic colors in the hierarchy proposed by Berlin and Kay.

Carey and Bartlett (1978) were interested in finding out how a new color word and its meaning are normally acquired and how this is affected by, and in turn affects, the semantic domain of colors. After initial assessment of preschool subjects' and matched controls' knowledge of colors on a wide range of tasks, subjects were introduced to a new color term (*chromium*) and its referent on several occasions. Between presentations they and their matched controls were retested to determine what they had learned about the new word and its referent and how the children integrated what they had learned into their lexicons. Carey and Bartlett found that if a first color word and its referent were already known, one or two isolated and brief exposures to a new color term were sufficient to affect children's naming of the color, and that children retained the knowledge sufficiently to build on it two months later. In addition, they documented a variety of strategies used by different children in integrating the new information into their lexicons.

As children's vocabularies grow, measuring vocabulary size and assessing children's word knowledge become very difficult (Miller & Wakefield, 1993). Should *cat* and *cats* be counted as two words? Should *walk, walks, walking,* and *walked* all be counted as a single word? Does a child who correctly uses the verb *run* and the noun *run* with reference to a baseball game also know how to refer appropriately to a *run* in her mother's stocking?

The difficulty of assessing children's semantic knowledge arises, of course, because children's semantic systems themselves are becoming more complex. Not only do children learn new words and new concepts, they also enrich and solidify their knowledge of known words by establishing multiple links among words and concepts.

For example, children learn that the words *cat* and *cats* refer to the same category of animate object, but differ in number, while the words *cats* and *books* share the feature *number* even though they refer to quite different objects. The words *walk, walks, walking,* and *walked* refer to similar actions that differ in tense or duration, while *eat* and *devour* refer to actions that differ in manner. *Compete, win,* and *lose* share some semantic components, but differ in the outcome each conveys. *Pain* and *pane* are linked phonologically, as are *pane, mane,* and *lane,* though each has a different referent. *Oak, spruce,* and *birch* are linked by virtue of their co-membership in the superordinate category *tree.* These types of connections among words and concepts form what are called **semantic networks.**

Although formation of semantic networks continues throughout the life span, there is evidence that children begin forming rudimentary semantic networks very early in development. Clark (1993), for example, notes that children often add several new words for one semantic domain all at once, as when one-year-old Damon learned *ant, bug,* and *ladybug* all in one week, and *frog, snake,* and *alligator* the next.

According to Bowerman (1978), children seek links, relationships, and conceptual wholes in everything they experience, including language. As a result, they add to their vocabularies not only words that will give them new communicative possibilities, but also synonyms that do not increase their communicative abilities. Other semantic links are evident in preschoolers' inappropriate use of certain words after they have learned the appropriate use. In such cases, Bowerman found elements of meaning shared by the misused word and the word called for in the context. An example of this phenomenon (appropriate use of a word interrupted by temporary inappropriate use) was given by two-year-old Christy, who said, "Daddy take his pants on" (p. 986) when previously in such cases she had used *put* instead of *take.* Both terms refer to actions that result in a change of location for an object, and Bowerman suggested that such substitutions can be interpreted most adequately as "incorrect choices among semantically related words that compete for selection in a particular speech context" (p. 979).

Another indication that words in children's vocabularies are becoming interconnected is developmental change that has been documented in children's **word associations.** Significantly, responses to such tasks have been shown to be indicative of other measures of linguistic sophistication (Brown & Berko, 1960). There are three general types of word association tasks that have been used. In **free-word-association** tasks, children are given a particular word and instructed to give the next word that comes to mind (see Palermo, 1971; Palermo & Jenkins, 1963). In **restricted-word-association** tasks, children are given additional semantic criteria for selecting responses; for example, the response must bear a particular relationship to the stimulus word, such as superordinate, opposite, or rhyming (see Riegel, Riegel, Quarterman, & Smith, 1968).

In **set tests,** children are given the name of a language category, such as "animals" or "furniture," and are asked to supply as many names of category members as they are able. On all three types of tasks, older individuals' responses represent a narrower, better-defined set than do those of younger children, and on set tests older children produce longer lists of group members. For example, Nelson (1974) found that eight- year-olds were able to supply nearly twice the number of responses of five-year-olds, and only the five-year-olds included "meat" and "ice cream" in the vegetable category and "wall" and "door" in the furniture category.

Young children respond to free-word-association tasks with words that are related in syntax to the stimulus word; that is, they give words that would typically follow the stimulus word in a normal sentence (Brown & Berko, 1960; Entwisle, 1966). For example, in response to the stimulus word *eat,* a child might say "lunch." In contrast, older individuals tend to respond with words that are of the same grammatical category as the stimulus word (e.g., *eat*—"drink"). Around age seven, children begin to respond with class-related words. While this trend in response pattern continues to evolve from first grade to college, it shows by far the greatest change between first and second grades. Explanations for the shift include general cognitive strategy shifts (Nelson, 1977), developmental changes in children's interpretation of the task, changes in knowledge of the features that define words (Lippman, 1971; McNeill, 1966), and cognitive reorganization that accompanies the acquisition of reading (Cronin, 1987).

Metalinguistic Development

The primary focus of this chapter is on children's development of semantic knowledge, in which words symbolize, or stand for, particular meanings. Once we know the meanings of words, we do not need to notice the words themselves in order to appreciate the information they carry. However, along with the development of semantic knowledge, children come to appreciate that language has potential greater than that of simple symbols. Children begin to notice words as objects, and later become able to manipulate them to learn to read and write and to accomplish a host of nonliteral ends such as using metaphors, creating puns, and using irony. These language uses depend on **metalinguistic awareness, or knowledge of the nature of language as an** object. Metalinguistic awareness develops gradually through the middle school years.

Before children can engage in flexible uses of words, they must have an implicit understanding that words are separable from their referents. Young children often consider the name of an object another of its intrinsic attributes. They believe, for instance, that if you called a horse *cow,* it might begin to moo. Later, children learn that words themselves are not inherent attributes of objects, which allows them to move beyond literal word use and adopt a metaphoric stance.

Once children understand that a word and its referent are separable, they can begin to reflect on the properties of words and objects separately. They learn that although words and their referents sometimes share properties, more often they do not. For example, *elephant* and *hippopotamus* are big words for big animals; however, other long words such as *mosquito* and *dragonfly* refer to very tiny insects. Similarly, while the sound of the words *slip, slide,* and *slink* convey a notion of smooth motion, the sounds of the words *crocus* and *sunset* suggest nothing of the beauty of their referents.

Children's ability to compare and contrast such properties *explicitly,* in a formal way, develops only gradually over a period of several years, but even very young children on occasion are able to appreciate and reflect upon the physical attributes of words (Chaney, 1992). For example, preschoolers can recognize and sometimes comment that different pronunciations of words do not alter their meanings (Leopold, 1948). Children as young as two or three also engage in spontaneous rhyming, which involves implicit comparison and matching of phonological sequences within words, and they recognize that some words include other words within them (e.g., *garden* includes *den*). Occasionally, children's awareness of phonological sequences, combined with their tendency to assume a relationship between form and meaning, may lead them to predict incorrect semantic correspondences between words that sound similar. Thus at four years of age, Phoebe, on the basis of her knowledge of *tomato,* believed that *tornadoes* were whirling masses of red air; and Polly, who knew the word *eagle,* wondered whether *beagle* referred to a kind of dog that could fly (Pease, 1986).

Many studies that aim to examine children's developing metalinguistic notions of the concept of "word" require that the child be able to verbalize such concepts. For example, in a seminal study of word awareness, Papandropoulou and Sinclair (1974) presented preschool and elementary school children with a variety of metalinguistic tasks, including one in which children were read a list of words, asked whether each was a word, and then asked for explanations for each response. The researchers observed improvement across the ages studied, both in children's recognition of words and in their ability to verbalize such concepts. Specifically, older children acknowledged both content and function words as words, while younger children sometimes rejected the latter; further, older children were more adept at articulating what constitutes a word.

It is likely, however, that well before children can demonstrate such explicit knowledge on demand, they have a rudimentary awareness of the nature of words. This view is supported, for instance, by a study by Bowey, Pratt, and Tunmer (1984), who found that preschoolers, and first- and second-graders benefited significantly from a brief training session in correctly identifying single words from lists including phrases and nonspeech sounds. Another study (Pease, 1986) that attempted to examine children's implicit awareness of the concept of "word" took a somewhat different approach in order to minimize performance demands. Children between the ages of four-and-a-half and ten years were simply asked to tell what their favorite words and favorite things were. Even at the youngest ages, most children differentiated between the two questions, though they were sometimes unable to explain their responses. A few preschoolers failed to differentiate the two concepts, naming favorite things in response to both questions. For example, one child's favorite word was *toys* because "they are fun to play with" and her favorite thing was *car,* again because "it's fun to play with." In the kindergarten group, some children were even able to articulate the reason why a particular word was their favorite (e.g., the word *ear* because "it sounds neat"). The ability to differentiate between the two questions and to articulate met-aliguistic aspects of words was even clearer at older ages, with children reporting favorite objects or activities (e.g., "swimming") for favorite things and giving words with interesting sound or spelling patterns (e.g., *petrified* or *Mississippi*) for favorite words. Furthermore, the oldest children reported that they and their friends had talked about words they liked, indicating that by the early school years children are actively and explicitly reflecting on and discussing words as objects.

Segmentation

Children's awareness of words in context has also been investigated. Researchers have studied the development of children's ability to segment a stream of speech into words, syllables, and phonemes. The ability to correctly segment at the word level, in particular, would facilitate mapping of spoken language onto written language. Although literate adults may find the identification of word units in spoken language a trivial task, in fact boundaries between words in a stream of speech are not identifiable on the basis of pauses or other acoustic features. Thus, children must depend on a variety of other cues and information about semantics and syntax in order to identify word boundaries. The age at which children are able to segment utterances into adult word units varies depending on how the task is presented and on what response is required of the child (cf. Ehri, 1975; Fox & Routh, 1975; Hardy, Stennet, & Smyth, 1973; Huttenlocher, 1964). Sometimes children are asked to count the words in a spoken utterance, tap out each word in a phrase or sentence, or represent each word with a token. Such tasks involve auditory memory and the coordination of a verbal or motoric response, as well as metalinguistic awareness. Coordinating the various elements of the task tends to be difficult for preschoolers. Tasks in which children are asked instead to repeat smaller and smaller "bits" of an utterance are somewhat easier (Fox & Routh, 1975).

A different technique was used by Huttenlocher (1964), who presented children with pairs of words and asked them either to reverse the members of the pair or to pause between them. The pairs of words that were least likely to occur together in normal speech (e.g., *peach–apple*) were the easiest for children to separate, while those that often occur together (e.g., *happy–birthday*) were more difficult. Huttenlocher concluded that children as young as four are aware of words, but that their awareness is strongly related to the context in which the words appear. It may be that successful accomplishment of such "simpler" segmentation tasks relies more on perceptual skills than on a conceptual awareness of words; alternatively, it may be that when extraneous task demands are reduced in this way, children are better able to demonstrate their awareness of words.

More recently, when Chaney (1989) looked at the developing metalinguistic awareness of word boundaries in children between the ages of four-and-a-half and six-and-a-half, she found that children first were able to recognize phrase boundaries, then syllable boundaries, and finally were able to segment according to word boundaries. When children were faced with unknown or more abstract words, they tended to revert to a phrase strategy or to substitute common, known words for the unknown ones. Some substitutions made in repeating the Pledge of Allegiance were "the night of states" instead of "the United States," "for witches stand" instead of "for which it stands," and "liver T" instead of "liberty." It is perhaps not surprising that children's first strategy is to segment at the phrasal level, since phrases are relatively self-contained units of meaning. Children's later segmenting at syllable and word boundaries may reflect their growing ability to attend to the physical, auditory properties of segments, rather than to semantic properties exclusively.

It is worth noting that most of these studies involved children who already had some experience with written language or who were in the process of learning to read. Because developmental change in children's word awareness tends to coincide with their beginning to read, researchers have been interested in exploring the role certain kinds of metalinguistic awareness may play in reading readiness and reading acquisition. Word segmentation skills in first-graders, for example, have been shown to be strong predictors of later reading success (Evans, Taylor, & Blum, 1979). Of course, the converse is also possible; experience with seeing words represented on paper may facilitate children's segmentation of the speech stream into adult word units. Tentative support for the latter is found in research by Kolinsky, Cary, and Morais (1987) with illiterate adults and adults who had only recently learned to read. When their subjects were asked to produce long and short words and to match spoken words of different lengths to written words, those with some reading experience were better able to perform the task than those without. Like young prereaders, adults without reading experience tended to produce long and short phrases, rather than words. This research suggests that literacy and experience with printed matter may promote awareness of certain physical aspects of words (see Chapter 10 for a discussion of the development of literacy).

Humor, Metaphor, and Irony

From very young ages, children can be observed to play with semantic elements in syntactic structures for humorous effect, as in: "Daddy's proud of you; Grandma's proud of you; Uncle David's proud of you; Hamburger not proud of you, ha ha!" (Horgan, 1981). Toddlers and preschoolers find word play such as rhyming and intentional nonsensical talk amusing and at times even hysterical, but delight in puns and riddles—like interest in favorite words—becomes particularly intense in the middle elementary school years. In fact, many humorous uses of language such as puns and riddles depend on the speaker's ability to separate different facets of language (cf. Horgan, 1981; McGhee, 1979; Schultz, 1976; Slobin, 1978). Thus, what some elementary teachers have dubbed "third-grade humor" is an overt sign that children are actively practicing and consolidating their metalinguistic skills.

In addition to using language for humorous effect, children also learn to use language in other nonliteral ways, such as metaphor and irony. Winner (1988) has studied the development of **metaphor**, which she says generally serves to clarify meaning, and **irony**, which is usually used to evaluate or criticize. Initially, the ability to understand metaphoric uses of language is important because it offers children an additional strategy for clarifying communication, both in production and in comprehension. Even very young children spontaneously use and understand certain types of metaphor for communicative purposes, though their use becomes much more fluent and less context-specific with age (Pearson, 1990). Later, in addition to its clarifying function, metaphor also begins to be used as an important tool in grasping new concepts in relatively unfamiliar areas of knowledge. Winner (1988) cites examples from a variety of fields (art, science, medicine,) in which analogy and metaphoric thinking greatly facilitated the generation of solutions to difficult problems. Both the clarifying and the problem-solving functions of metaphoric language and thinking continue to be crucial throughout the life span.

Using and understanding irony involves appreciating that words and phrases not only can have meanings different from their literal ones, but that the meaning the speaker intends to convey can in fact be precisely the opposite of what the surface meaning would suggest. Irony is most commonly used to express **sarcasm** (that is, the intent to criticize or insult). Adults rely both on contextual cues and on intonational cues in interpreting sarcasm. Thus if a speaker comments, "Nice catch," after a spectacularly clumsy miss, adult listeners will consider a nonliteral, or sarcastic interpretation even if the comment is made in a neutral tone of voice. Children, on the other hand, appear to be much more sensitive to intonational than to contextual cues (Capelli, Nakagawa, & Madden, 1990). Thus, despite the blatant mismatch between context and literal meaning, they might fail to interpret the "Nice catch" comment as sarcastic if it were expressed without the typical mocking intonation. Children younger than about eight rarely understand sarcasm even when intonational cues are present.

One first-grader we know got off the school bus with a big smile to report that a much-respected third-grader thought his new notebook was really neat. When asked how he knew the older child was so impressed with the new possession, the first-grader promptly replied, "because when I showed it to him he said, 'Big deal!'" Irony and sarcasm are probably other areas of metalinguistic awareness in which verbal interaction with peers provides the young language learner with important data and a forum in which to practice his developing communicative skills.

Word Definitions

Defining a word involves metalinguistic skills as well as semantic knowledge. Children's ability to use linguistic context to deduce the meanings of new words was studied by Werner and Kaplan (1950). In this landmark study, children were presented with a number of sentences with a nonsense word in the place of a key word (e.g., "The painter used a *corplum* to mix his paints" or "A wet *corplum* does not burn"). The children were to figure out the meanings of the nonsense words from their linguistic contexts. Werner and Kaplan found age-related differences in the strategies children used to perform the task. For instance, five-year-olds, who tended to fuse the meaning of the word with the meaning of the sentence, might define *corplum* by saying, "A corplum is wet and painters use it," whereas an eleven-year-old might say, "A corplum is a kind of stick!"

Defining a word involves metalinguistic skills as well as semantic knowledge. With development, children become better able to define words as semantically unique by including critical types of information and using different approaches to organize it. For example, during the early school years children's definitions are concrete (descriptions of the referent's appearance or function), personal, and incidental (Snow, 1990). Through the elementary school years, these are gradually joined by abstract types of responses: synonyms, explanations, and specifications of categorical relationships (Al-Issa, 1969; Litowitz, 1977; Wolman & Baker, 1965). Swartz and Hall (1972) compared children's word definitions and their performance on a variety of tasks involving relational concepts. They found that children who were least able to consider relational concepts favored *functional* definitions, whereas older children (ages nine to eleven), who were most able to consider relational concepts, gave a majority of *abstract* definitions. Wehren, DeLisi, and Arnold (1981) found a developmental progression in word definitions among children aged five to eleven and college students, beginning with an emphasis on personal experience and moving toward information of a more general, socially shared nature. Snow (1990) has shown that knowledge of the conventional form for good definitions (the definitional genre), combined with frequent opportunities to practice hearing and giving definitions, are necessary for the development of adultlike definitional skills.

A Lifelong Enterprise

Semantic development continues apace throughout the life span. Not only do we as adults continue to add new words to our lexicons, but we also continue to fine-tune the extensions of old words in response to widening experience and to social and cultural changes in our linguistic community. Reflection on and analysis of language result in continual lexical reorganization, a flexibility that is essential if we are to use our language in the most adaptive and effective way to address a wide variety of communicative tasks throughout the life span.

Summary

The relation between words and their referents is an arbitrary, symbolic one, defined by social convention. Thus, learning word meanings involves learning how one's own language community labels the physical and mental world. Developmental theorists suggest that very young children begin with certain predispositions, or principles, that help them quickly make initial word-to-referent mappings. For example, children may assume that words refer to whole objects, rather than to their parts, and that a single object can have only one name. Feedback from more competent speakers allows children to confirm or disprove their initial hypotheses and gradually make their mappings conform to those of their speech community.

Children's early vocabularies typically include more nouns than verbs or function words, perhaps because the referents of nouns are more concrete and more easily identifiable, or perhaps because they are more common in the speech addressed to young children. Unconventional word-to-meaning mappings (overextensions and underextensions) in children's early speech may reflect processing limitations such as retrieval errors, underlying conceptual differences, or even analogical use of limited vocabulary. Even very young children use language creatively to draw analogies, make jokes, and to invent their own words in systematic ways.

Many features of adult speech to young children are thought to facilitate children's semantic development. Slow, clear enunciation and exaggerated intonation may help children segment the speech stream and identify new words. Talk about the here and now and labeling of objects at the basic level may also simplify the mapping task.

As they get older, children not only continue to acquire new words and to learn new meanings for familiar words, but they also make connections among words. They learn, among other things, which words are similar in meaning, which contrast, which are subordinate to others, and which are phonologically related. In addition to semantic knowledge of words, children begin to develop the metalinguistic understanding that words themselves have properties that can be reflected on and discussed.

Key Words

basic level category	compound word
classical concept	constraints
color term	core group

deictic terms
derived word
focal colors
folk etymology
free-word association
irony
kinship terms
metalinguistic development
metalinguistic awareness
metaphor
novel name-nameless
   category principle
ontological categories
ostension
overextension
preferential looking paradigm
principle of contrast

principle of mutual exclusivity
principles
probabilistic concept
productivity
prototypes
referent
restricted-word association
sarcasm
semantic development
semantic feature
semantic network
semantic transparency
set test
shape bias
simplicity
underextension
word associations

Suggested Projects

1. Show adults and kindergarten children pictures of different kinds of birds and other flying creatures (e.g., bat, pterodactyl). Ask them to rank the pictures in order of bird-likeness. Compare the rankings of the adults and children. Did all the adults agree in their rankings, or were there fuzzy category boundaries?

2. Choose a passage of very technical language (e.g., legal document or technical manual). Practice reading it aloud until you can do it smoothly; then tape-record yourself reading it. Have five friends listen to the tape and write down what they hear. Examine their dictation samples to see if there are any incorrect segmentations.

3. Tape-record half-hour speech samples of a three-year-old and a five-year-old at play. Compare the topics they include and the words they use. What similarities and differences do you note?

4. Find a children's picture book with few or no words. Ask a parent of a child eighteen to twenty-four months old to spend ten or fifteen minutes using the book with the child. Ask a parent of a three-and-a-half-year-old to four-year-old child to do the same thing. Record and compare the words the parents use with the two children.

5. Ask children of different ages to tell their favorite words and things, and explain their choices. Compare their choices and explanations.

6. Ask children of different ages to define what *words* are.

7. Ask children of different ages to tell you what particular words mean. Include some words with multiple meanings, such as *cold*.

8. Ask a few children to think of specific referents, such as *dog*, and tell what they "see."

9. Tell children of different ages a sentence with a new word in it, and then ask what the word means.

Suggested Readings

Anglin, J. (1993). Vocabulary development: A morphological analysis. *Monographs of the Society for Research in Child Development, 58,* no. 10.

Au, T. K. (1990). Children's use of information in word learning. *Journal of Child Language, 17,* 393–416.

Bates, E., Marchman, V. Thal, D., Fenson, L., Dale, P., Reznick, S., Reilly, J., & Hartung, J. (1994). Developmental and stylistic variation in the composition of early vocabulary. *Journal of Child Language, 21,* 85–123.

Clark. E. V. (1993). *The lexicon in acquisition.* Cambridge, UK: Cambridge University Press.

Golinkoff, R., Mervis, C., & Hirsh-Pasek, K. (1994). Early object labels: The case for a developmental lexical principles framework. *Journal of Child Language, 21,* 125–155.

Haviland, S. E., & Clark, E. V. (1974). "This man's father is my father's son": A study of the acquisition of English kin terms. *Journal of Child Language, 1,* 23–47.

Mervis, C. B., & Mervis, C. A. (1982). Leopards are kitty-cats: Object labeling by mothers for their thirteen-month-olds. *Child Development, 53,* 267–273.

Nelson, K. (1974). Variations in children's concepts by age and category. *Child Development, 45,* 577–584.

Tunmer, W. E., Pratt, C., & Harriman, M. L. (1984). *Metalinguistic awareness in children.* Berlin: Springer-Verlag.

Werner, H., & Kaplan, E. (1950). Development of word meaning through verbal context: An experiment study. *Journal of Psychology, 29,* 251–257.

Winner, E. (1988). *The point of words: Children's understanding of metaphor and irony.* Cambridge, MA: Harvard University Press.

References

Aitchison, J. (1987). *Words in the mind: An introduction to the mental lexicon.* Oxford: Basil Blackwell.

Al-Issa, I. (1969). The development of word definitions in children. *Journal of Genetic Psychology, 114,* 25–28.

Andrick, G. R., & Tager-Flusberg, H. (1986). The acquisition of colour terms. *Journal of Child Language, 13,* 119–134.

Anglin, J. (1977). *Word, object, and conceptual development.* New York: Norton.

Anglin, J. (1978). From reference to meaning. *Child Development, 49,* 969–976.

Anglin, J. (1995). Classifying the world through language: Functional relevance, cultural significance, and category name learning. *International Journal of Intercultureal Relations, 19,* 161–181.

Au, T. K., & Glusman, M. (1990). The principle of mutual exclusivity in word learning: to honor or not to honor? *Child Development 61,* 1474–1490.

Baldwin, D. (1991). Infants' contribution to the achievement of joint reference. *Child Development, 62,* 875–890.

Bartlett, E. J. (1977). The acquisition of the meaning of color terms: A study of lexical development. In R. Campbell & P. Smith (Eds.), *Recent advances in the psychology of language* (Vol. 4a, pp. 89–108). New York: Plenum Press.

Bates, E., Marchman, V., Thal, D., Fenson, L., Dale, P., Reznick, S., Reilly, J., & Hartung, J. (1994). Developmental and stylistic variation in the composition of early vocabulary. *Journal of Child Language, 21,* 85–123.

Becker, J. (1994). Sneak-shoes, sworders, and nose-beards: A case study of lexical innovation. *First Language, 14,* 195–211.

Beeghly, M., Bretherton, I., & Mervis, C. (1986). Mothers' internal state language to toddlers: The socialization of psychological understanding. *British Journal of Developmental Psychology, 4,* 247–260.

Benedict, H. (1979). Early lexical development: Comprehension and production. *Journal of Child Language, 6,* 183–200.

Berko, J. (1958). The child's learning of English morphology. *Word, 14,* 150–177.

Berlin, B., & Kay, P. (1969). *Basic color terms: Their universality and evolution.* Berkeley: University of California Press.

Bloom, L., & Lahey, M. (1978). *Language development and language disorders.* New York: Wiley.

Bloomfield, L. (1933). *Language.* New York: Henry Holt.

Bowerman, M. (1978). Systematizing semantic knowledge: Changes over time in the child's organization of word meaning. *Child Development, 49,* 977–987.

Bowey, J. A., Pratt, C., & Tunmer, W. E. (1984). Development of children's understanding of the metalinguistic term "word." *Journal of Educational Psychology, 76,* 500–512.

Brown, R. (1968). *Words and things.* New York: Free Press.

Brown, R., & Berko, J. (1960). Word association and the acquisition of grammar. *Child Development, 31,* 1–14.

Callanan, M. A. (1985). How parents label objects for young children: The role of input in the acquisition of category hierarchies. *Child Development, 56,* 508–523.

Capelli, C., Nakagawa, N., & Madden, C. (1990). How children understand sarcasm: The role of context and intonation. *Child Development, 61,* 1824–1841.

Carabine, B. (1991). Fuzzy boundaries and the extension of object words. *Journal of Child Language, 18,* 355–372.

Carey, S., & Bartlett, E. (1978, August). Acquiring a single new word. *Papers and Reports on Child Language Development, 15,* 17–29.

Chaney, C. (1989). I pledge a legiance to the flag: Three studies in word segmentation. *Applied Psycholinguistics, 10,* 261–282.

Chaney, C. (1992). Language development, matalinguistic skills, and print awareness in three-year-old children. *Applied Psycholinguistics, 13,* 485–514.

Chapman, K. L., Leonard, L. B., & Mervis, C. B. (1986). The effect of feedback on young children's inappropriate word usage. *Journal of Child Language, 13,* 101–117.

Charles-Luce, J., & Luce, P. A. (1990). Similarity neighborhoods of words in young children's lexicons. *Journal of Child Language, 17,* 205–215.

Clark, E. V. (1974). Some aspects of the conceptual basis for first language acquisition. In R. L. Schiefelbusch & L. L. Lloyd (Eds.), *Language perspectives—Acquisition, retardation, and intervention.* Baltimore: University Park Press.

Clark, E. V. (1978). Strategies for communicating. *Child Development, 49,* 953–959.

Clark, E. V. (1981). Lexical innovations: How children learn to create new words. In W. Deutsch (Ed.), *The child's construction of language.* London: Academic Press.

Clark, E. V. (1982). The young word maker: A case study of innovations in the child's lexicon. In E. Wanner & L. R. Gleitman (Eds.), *Language acquisition: The state of the art.* New York: Cambridge University Press.

Clark, E. V. (1987). The principle of contrast: A constraint on language acquisition. In B. MacWhinney (Ed.), *Mechanisms of language acquisition.* Hillsdale, NJ: Lawrence Erlbaum.

Clark, E. V. (1993). *The lexicon in acquisition.* Cambridge, UK: Cambridge University Press.

Clark, E. V., & Sengul, C. J. (1978). Strategies in the acquisition of deixish. *Journal of Child Language, 5,* 457–475.

Cronin, V. (1987). Word association and reading. Paper presented at the meeting of the Society for Research in Child Development, Baltimore, MD.

Cross, T. G. (1977). Mothers' speech adjustments: The contributions of selected child listener variables. In C. Ferguson & C. Snow (Eds.), *Talking to children: Language input and acquisition.* Cambridge, UK: Cambridge University Press.

Dale, P. S., Bates, E., Reznick, J. S., & Morisset, C. (1989). The validity of a parent report instrument of child language at twenty months. *Journal of Child Language, 16,* 239–250.

Danziger, K. (1957). The child's understanding of kinship terms: A study in the development of relational concepts. *Journal of Genetic Psychology, 91,* 213–232.

deVilliers, P. A., & deVilliers, J. G. (1974). On this, that, and the other: Nonegocentrism in very young children. *Journal of Experimental Child Psychology, 18,* 438–447.

Dunn, J., Bretherton, I., & Munn, R. (1987). Conversations about feeling states between mothers and their young children. *Developmental Psychology, 23,* 132–139.

Ehri, L. C. (1975). Word consciousness in readers and prereaders. *Journal of Educational Psychology, 67,* 204–212.

Entwisle, D. R. (1966). *Word association responses of young children.* Baltimore: Johns Hopkins University Press.

Evans, M., Taylor, N., & Blum, I. (1979). Children's written language awareness and its relationship to reading acquisition. *Journal of Reading Behavior, 11,* 7–19.

Ferguson, C., & Farwell, C. (1975). Words and sounds in early language acquisition: English initial consonants in the first 50 words. *Language, 51,* 419–439.

Fernald, A. (1992) Meaningful melodies in mothers' speech to infants. In Papousek, H., Jurgens, U., and Papousek, M. (Eds.). *Origins and development of nonverbal vocal communication: Evolutionary, comparative, and methodological aspects.* Cambridge, UK: Cambridge University Press.

Fernald, A., & Mazzie, C. (1991). Prosody and focus in speech to infants and adults. *Developmental Psychology, 27,* 209–221.

Fox, F., & Routh, D. K. (1975). Analyzing spoken language into words, syllables, and phonemes: A developmental study. *Journal of Psycholinguistic Research, 4,* 331–342.

Gentner, D. (1983, February). Nouns and verbs. Symposium presented at the meeting of the New England Child Language Association, Tufts University Medford, MA.

Gentner, D. (1988). Cognitive determinism: Object reference and relational reference. Paper presented at the Boston University Child Language Conference, Boston, MA.

Gleason, J. Berko, & Ely, R. (1996). What color is the cat? Color words in parent–child conversations. Paper presented at the International Association for the Study of Child Language, Istanbul, 1996.

Goldfield, B. (1993). Noun bias in maternal speech to one-year-olds. *Journal of Child Language, 20,* 85–99.

Golinkoff, R., Hirsh-Pasek, K., Cauley, K., & Gordon, P. (1987). The eyes have it: Lexical and syntactic comprehension in a new paradigm. *Journal of Child Language, 14,* 23–46.

Golinkoff, R., Mervis, C., & Hirsh-Pasek, K. (1994). Early object labels: The case for a developmental lexical principles framework. *Journal of Child Language, 21,* 125–155.

Golinkoff, R., Shuff-Bailey, M., Olguin, R., & Ruan, W. (1995). Young children extend novel words at the basic level: Evidence for the principle of categorical scope. *Developmental Psychology, 31,* 494–507.

Hall, D. (1994a). Semantic constraints on word learning: Proper names and adjectives. *Child Development, 65,* 1299–1317.

Hall, D. (1994b). How mothers teach basic-level and situation-restricted count nouns. *Journal of Child Language, 21,* 391–414.

Hardy, M., Stennet, R. G., & Smyth, P. C. (1973). Auditory segmentation and auditory blending in relation to beginning reading. *The Alberta Journal of Educational Research, 19,* 144–158.

Haviland, S. E., & Clark, E. V. (1974). "This man's father is my father's son": A study of the acquisition of English kin terms. *Journal of Child Language, 1,* 23–47.

Hoek, D., Ingram, D., & Gibson, D. (1986). Some possible causes of children's early word overextensions. *Journal of Child Language, 13,* 477–494.

Horgan, D. (1981). Learning to tell jokes: A case study of metalinguistic abilities. *Journal of Child Language, 8,* 217–227.

Hudson, J., & Nelson, K. (1984). Play with language: Overextensions as analogies. *Journal of Child Language, 11,* 337–346.

Huttenlocher, J. (1964). Children's language: Word-phrase relationship. *Science, 143,* 264–265.

Huttenlocher, J. (1974). The origins of language comprehension. In R. L. Solso (Ed.), *Theories in cognitive psychology.* New York: Erlbaum.

Kolinsky, R., Cary, L., & Morais, J. (1987). Awareness of words as phonological entities: The role of literacy. *Applied Psycholinguistics, 8,* 223–232.

Landau, B., Smith, L., & Jones, S. (1988). The importance of shape in early lexical learning. *Cognitive Development, 3,* 199–321.

Lashley, K. S. (1954). The problem of serial order in behavior. In L. A. Jeffress (Ed.), *Cerebral mechanisms in behavior.* New York: Wiley.

Leonard, L. B., Schwartz, R., Folger, M., Newhoff, M., & Wilcox, M. (1979). Children's imitations of lexical items. *Child Development, 50,* 19–27.

Leonard, L. B., Schwartz, R. G., Morris, B., & Chapman, K. (1981). Factors influencing early lexical acquisition: Lexical orientation and phonological composition. *Child Development, 52,* 882–887.

Leopold, W. (1948). Semantic learning in infant language. *Word, 4,* 179.

Leopold, W. (1970). *Speech development of a bilingual child* (Vols. 1–4). New York: AMS Press.

Lippman, M. Z. (1971). Correlates of contrast word associations: Developmental trends. *Journal of Verbal Learning and Verbal Behavior, 10,* 392–399.

Litowitz, B. (1977). Learning to make definitions. *Journal of Child Language, 4,* 289–304.

Locke, J. L. (1993) *The child's path to spoken language.* Cambridge, MA: Harvard University Press.

Macnamara, J. (1972). Cognitive basis of language learning in infants. *Psychological Review, 79,* 1–13.

Macnamara, J. (1982). *Names for things: A study of human learning.* Cambridge, MA: MIT/ Bradford.

Markman, E. (1987). How children constrain the possible meanings of words. In U. Neisser (Ed.), *Concepts and conceptual development: Ecological and intellectual factors in categorization.* Cambridge, UK: Cambridge University Press.

Markman, E. M., & Wachtel, G. F. (1988). Children's use of mutual exclusivity to constrain the meanings of words. *Cognitive Psychology, 20,* 121–157.

McGhee, P. (1979). *Humor: Its origin and development.* San Francisco: Freeman.

McNeill, D. (1966). A study of word association. *Journal of Verbal Learning and Verbal Behavior, 5,* 548–557.

Mervis, C. B., & Mervis, C. A. (1982). Leopards are kitty-cats: Object labeling by mothers for their thirteen-month-olds. *Child Development, 53,* 267–273.

Mervis, C. B., & Mervis, C. A. (1988). Role of adult input in young children's category evolution. I. An observational study. *Journal of Child Language, 15,* 257–272.

Miller, G. & Wakefield, P. (1993). On Anglin's analysis of vocabulary growth. *Monographs of the Society for Research in Child Development, 58,* 167–175.

Morris, C. W (1946). *Signs, language, and behavior.* New York: Prentice-Hall.

Naigles, L., & Gelman, S. (1995). Overextensions in comprehension and production revisited: Preferential looking in a study of *dog, cat,* and *cow. Journal of Child Language, 22,* 19–46.

Nelson, K. (1974). Variations in children's concepts by age and category. *Child Development, 45,* 577–584.

Nelson, K. (1977). The syntagmatic-paradigmatic shift revisited: A review of research and theory. *Psychological Bulletin, 84,* 93–116.

Nelson, K., Benedict, H., Gruendel, J., & Rescorla, L. (1977). Lessons from early lexicons. Paper presented at the meeting of the Society for Research in Child Development, New Orleans.

Newport, E. L. (1975). Motherese: The speech of mothers to young children (Tech. Rep. No. 52). San Diego: University of California, Center for Human Information Processing.

Ninio, A., & Bruner, J. (1978). The achievement and antecedents of labeling. *Journal of Child Language, 5,* 1–14.

Palermo, D. S. (1971). Characteristics of word association responses obtained from children in grades one through four. *Developmental Psychology, 5*(l), 118–123.

Palermo, D. S., & Jenkins, J. J. (1963). *Word association norms: Grade school through college.* Minneapolis: University of Minnesota Press.

Papandropoulou, I., & Sinclair, H. (1974). What is a word? *Human Development, 17,* 241–258.

Pearson, B. Z. (1990). The comprehension of metaphor by preschool children. *Journal of Child Language, 17,* 185–203.

Pease, D. M. (1986). The development of semantic and metalinguistic knowledge. Unpublished doctoral dissertation, Boston University.

Phillips, J. R. (1973). Syntax and vocabulary of mothers' speech to young children: Age and sex comparisons. *Child Development, 44,* 182–185.

Piaget, J. (1928). *Judgment and reasoning in the child.* London: Routledge and Kegan Paul.

Poulin-Dubois, D. (1995). Object parts and the acquisition of the meaning of names. In K. Nelson & Z. Réger (Eds.), *Children's language, v.8.* Hillsdale, NJ: Lawrence Erlbaum.

Rescorla, L. A. (1980). Overextension in early language development. *Journal of Child Language, 7,* 321–335.

Rescorla, L. A. (1981). Category development in early language. *Journal of Child Language, 8,* 225–238.

Riegel, K. F., Riegel, R. M., Quarterman, C. J., & Smith, H. E. (1968). An analysis of difference in word meaning and semantic structure between four educational levels. *Human Development, 11,* 92–106.

Rosch, E. (1973). Natural categories. *Cognitive Psychology, 4,* 328–350.

Rosch, E., Mervis, C. B., Gray, W. D., Johnson, D. M., & Boyes-Braem, P. (1976). Basic objects in natural categories. *Cognitive Psychology, 8,* 382–439.

Sachs, J., Brown, R., & Salerno, R. (1976). Adults' speech to children. In W. von Raffler Engel and Y. Lebrun (Eds.), *Baby talk and infant speech.* Lisse, The Netherlands: Swets and Zeitlinger.

Schultz, T. (1976). A cognitive-developmental analysis of humor. In A. J. Chapman & M. C. Foot (Eds.), *Humor and laughter: Theory, research, and applications.* New York: Wiley.

Schwartz, R. G., & Leonard, L. B. (1982). Do children pick and choose? An examination of phonological selection and avoidance in early lexical acquisition. *Journal of Child Language, 9,* 319–336.

Shatz, M., & Gelman, R. (1973). The development of communication skills: Modifications in the speech of young children as a function of the listener. *Monographs of the Society for Research in Child Development, 38* (No. 152).

Slobin, D. I. (1978). A case study of early language awareness. In A. Sinclair, R. J. Jarvella, & W. J. Levelt (Eds.), *The child's conception of language.* New York: Wiley.

Smith, C. A., & Sachs, J. (1990). Cognition and the verb lexicon in early lexical development. *Applied Psycholinguistics, 11,* 409–424.

Smith, E. E., & Medin, D. L. (1981). *Categories and concepts.* Cambridge, MA: Harvard University Press.

Snow, C. (1972). Mothers' speech to children learning language. *Child Development, 43,* 549–585.

Snow, C. (1990). The development of definitional skill. *Journal of Child Language, 17,* 697–710.

Soja, N. (1994). Young children's concept of color and its relation to the acquisition of color words. *Child Development, 65,* 918–937.

Stoel-Gammon, C., & Cooper, J. A. (1984). Patterns of early lexical and phonological development. *Journal of Child Language, 11,* 247–271.

Swartz, K., & Hall, A. (1972). Development of relational concepts and word definitions in children five through eleven. *Child Development, 43,* 239–244.

Thompson, J. R., & Chapman, R. S. (1977). Who is "Daddy" revisited: The status of two-year-olds' overextended words in use and comprehension. *Journal of Child Language, 4,* 359–375.

Tichener, G. B. (1909). *Lectures on the experimental psychology of the thought processes.* New York: Macmillan.

Tiedemann, D. (1787). Über die Entwicklung der Seelenfähigkeiten bei Kindern. *Hessiche Bectragzur Gelehrsamkeit und Kunst.* Reprinted in English in A. Bar-Adon & W. Leopold (Eds.). (1971). Child language: A Book of readings. Englewood Cliffs, NJ: Prentice-Hall.

Tingley, E., Gleason, J. Berko, & Hooshyar, N. (1994). Mothers' lexicon of internal state words in speech to children with Down syndrome and to nonhandicapped children at mealtime. *Journal of Communication Disorders, 27,* 135–155.

Vygotsky, L. S. (1962). *Thought and language.* Cambridge, MA: MIT Press.

Webb, P. A., & Abrahamson, A. A. (1976). Stages of egocentrism in children's use of "this" and "that": A different point of view. *Journal of Child Language, 3,* 349–367.

Wehren, A., DeLisi, R., & Arnold, M. (1981). The development of noun definition. *Journal of Child Language, 8,* 165–175.

Werner, H., & Kaplan, E. (1950). Development of word meaning through verbal context: An experiment study. *Journal of Psychology, 29,* 251–257.

Winner, E. (1988). *The point of words: Children's understanding of metaphor and irony.* Cambridge, MA: Harvard University Press.

Wolman, R. N., & Baker, E. N. (1965). A developmental study of word definitions. *Journal of Genetic Psychology, 107,* 159–166.

Woodward, A., Markman, E., & Fitzsimmons, C. (1994). Rapid word learning in 13- and 18-month-olds. *Developmental Psychology, 30,* 553–566.

Chapter Five

Putting Words Together: Morphology and Syntax in the Preschool Years

Helen Tager-Flusberg, *University of Massachusetts at Boston*

Introduction

After months of coaxing and prompting the meaningless babbles of their babies, parents are finally rewarded when the first word is produced. Several weeks after this important milestone is duly recorded, vocabulary begins to grow quite rapidly, as new words are learned daily. At this initial stage young children use their words in a variety of contexts, most frequently to label objects or to interact socially, but always limit their messages by speaking one word at a time. Still, parents and children together delight in showing off these earliest linguistic accomplishments that mark the beginning of the journey toward full mastery of language.

Within a few months, usually in the latter half of the second year, children reach the next important milestone: They begin putting words together to form the first "sentences." This new stage marks a crucial turning point, for even the simplest two-word utterances show evidence of **syntax**; that is, the child combines words to create sentences following certain rules rather than in random fashion. One of the remarkable features about the development of syntactic rules is that it seems to take place almost unnoticed, with no explicit instruction. Parents who quite consciously and conscientiously teach their children new concepts and words never presume to teach syntax. They focus more on *what* the child is saying rather than *how* the child says it (Brown & Hanlon, 1970).

Even though parents and others have essentially ignored the child's use and occasional misuse of syntactic rules, child language researchers and linguists have studied that usage closely all over the world. Years of careful and painstaking research have yielded a detailed, descriptive picture of the course of syntactic development in

English and other languages, although the mechanisms that account for these accomplishments are still being hotly debated (see Chapter 7). In this chapter, we describe the main stages of syntactic development that take place during the preschool years, focusing on the order in which various constructions are acquired. At each stage we are concerned with extracting the universal and invariant features of children's language and characterizing the underlying knowledge of linguistic rules and categories that fit the language at that point in development.

The Nature of Syntactic Rules

Much of our understanding of the nature of syntactic rules has come from linguists who have been concerned primarily with characterizing the rules that underlie the well-formed sentences of adult language users—the natural end point of the acquisition process. The most influential linguistic framework is the one developed by Noam Chomsky, called the theory of **universal grammar,** or UG. Chomsky began developing this framework in 1957, but it has undergone several revisions since. The current version is known as **government and binding theory,** or GB (Chomsky, 1981, 1982). Because this theory has had such a significant influence on research on grammatical development, especially in recent years, we shall first describe briefly some of the major concepts and characteristics of this linguistic premise.

According to Chomsky, the goals of any theory of grammar, such as universal grammar, are that it is compatible with the grammars of all the world's languages (the goal of **universality**), and that it must, in principle, be compatible with the fact that children worldwide acquire the grammar of their language within a few short years, usually with little or no explicit training or correction (the goal of **learnability**). GB theory is a theory of language knowledge; essentially, it is a theory of how we represent language as a set of principles in our mind. Chomsky believes that our mental representation of grammar is autonomous of other cognitive systems, which means that the principles and rules of grammar are not shared with other cognitive systems but are in fact unique and highly specialized.

The central tenet of GB theory is that there are several components of the grammar that are linked at different levels of representation. Figure 5.1 provides a simplified view of the main components. Of key interest are the two levels: **d-structure,** which captures the underlying relationships between subject and object in a sentence (the basic unit of grammar); and **s-structure,** which captures the surface linear arrangements of words in a sentence. In order to see why these two levels are necessary, consider the following sentences:

> John is easy to please.
> John is eager to please.

Both sentences have virtually the same s-structures:

> noun–verb–adjective–infinitive verb.

However, they mean quite different things. The subject of the verb "to please" is John in the second sentence, but someone else in the first. This difference in the underlying grammatical relationships of subject, predicate, and so forth would be captured by very different d-structures. From a developmental point of view, we must ask the question of how children come to grasp the underlying grammatical relations of sentences they hear (d-structures), when they are only presented with s-structures.

Figure 5.1 also shows that each level, s-structure and d-structure, has several components. The s-structure has two parts: **phonetic form,** which is the actual sound structure of the sentence; and **logical form,** which captures the meaning of sentences (this component connects the grammar to other aspects of cognition). The d-structure also has two parts: the **phrase structure rules,** which capture the basic subject/predicate structure of a sentence; and the *lexicon,* which specifies a number of important features (morphophonological, syntactic) for each lexical item in a sentence. Together, the lexicon and the phrase structure rules generate the d-structure of a sentence.

The phrase structures are often represented in "tree-diagrams" of the sort you see in Figure 5.2. They capture the underlying relationships of parts or *phrases* of the sentence, including *noun phrases, verb phrases, adjectival phrases,* etc. The phrase structure of a sentence also includes some additional syntactic elements, such as *complementizers (that, what),* which introduces each sentence, and an *inflectional* category, which holds the auxiliary verb (*do, will, may,* etc.) and carries information about tense. Thus the basic structure of the sentence is organized in the d-structure by the phrase structure rules. And within these phrases, we see that there are two important types of *categories.* One type is called a **lexical category,** headed by lexical forms such as nouns or

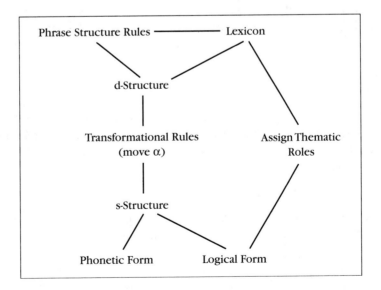

Figure 5.1

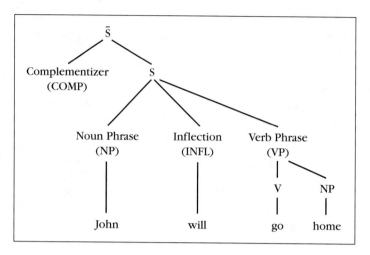

Figure 5.2

verbs; the other is called a **functional category**, which is a grammatical category, such as inflectional (INFL) or complementizer (COMP), as shown in Figure 5.2. This distinction plays an important part in current theories of grammatical development (e.g., Radford, 1990).

The lexicon provides the specific "words" or lexical items that get inserted at the end of the phrase structure trees. The lexicon contains information for each item about its syntactic category (noun, verb, adjective, etc.), much like a dictionary. It also contains information about what kinds of sentence structures the item requires, which is especially important for verbs. Consider the following set of verbs:

    run

    see

    put

The lexicon would include different information for each verb because they all appear in different sentence structures, or *argument structure.* Thus the verb *run* only requires a subject; it does not require an object, but it could take a location as an optional argument:

    John runs (to the store).

The verb *see* requires both a subject and an object, and it can take as an object either a simple noun phrase or a complete sentence:

    John sees Mary (writing her book).

The verb *put* not only requires a subject and object, but also needs a location specified:

John put the book on the shelf.

This information about the argument structure of different verbs is all contained in the lexicon, and is critical in organizing appropriate phrase structures. In addition to required arguments, additional optional phrases may also be added to other phrases in a sentence. For example,

John put the book on the shelf *last night.*

This optional phrase is referred to as an *adjunct.*

The d-structure is connected to the s-structure by a rule that reorders the elements of the phrase structure into the linear arrangement of the surface form. This rule, called the **transformational rule,** is extremely general—"move any category anywhere"—which allows elements to get moved around. This movement rule is important in English—for example, in creating questions (as in the example in Figure 5.3) or passive constructions. Because the transformational rule is so general, the grammar also needs to have a set of rules, or *constraints,* on which elements may be moved and which may not, as well as where they may be moved to. Many of these restrictions are included in the numerous subtheories that form a part of the GB framework, but we will not go into these here. Some constraints are universal and apply to all languages; some are specific to each language (e.g., the English question-formation rule that moves the *wh-* word to the beginning of the sentence).

The lexicon is also connected to the logical form component of s-structure (see Figure 5.1) via the assignment of **thematic roles** (also called **semantic roles** in other

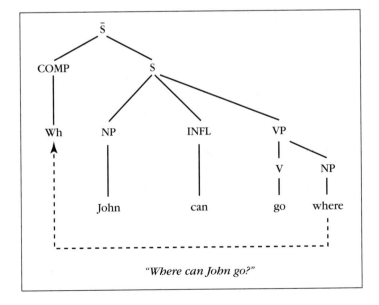

Figure 5.3

linguistic systems). This assigns to each of the main noun phrases a role in the sentence like agent, patient, recipient, and location:

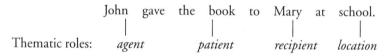

All these components and rule systems are considered to be universal in UG. The grammar also has a system for handling the kind of syntactic and morphological variations that exist across languages of the world. UG includes a set of principles that vary as **parameters.** They operate one way for some languages and another way for other languages. These parameters are conceived of as a set of switches, with several settings (typically two) on each switch. In theory, at least, each language's grammar is captured by a unique combination of switch settings on all the main parameters. This is one of the exciting new ideas in UG, because it addresses the goal of universality, but so far not many parameters have been well worked out. It is also an important idea for researchers of language development, because one hypothesis that has been proposed is that in each child UG starts off with its collection of parameters. As a child is exposed to her native language, the evidence from this input is used to guide which way the switches on each parameter should be set. Thus, the parameter setting hypothesis also addresses the goal of learnability (Meisel, 1995).

One example of a parameter is called the *null-subject parameter* (sometimes also called *pro-drop*). In English, every sentence is required to have an explicit subject; however, languages such as Italian or Spanish allow sentences to drop their subjects in the s-structure. So, for example, one can say in Italian:

Sta piovendo. (Is raining).

For this sentence to be grammatical in English, we must add an *It* as the subject, although the pronoun does not refer to anything at all. This kind of pronoun is called an *expletive,* and only languages that require subjects also have expletive pronouns. There are other differences between Italian and English that all covary under the null-subject parameter. In this way language variation is captured by an economical system that considers under a single parameter a range of correlated syntactic features. We shall see later in this chapter how this idea of parameters, especially the null-subject parameter, has motivated some interesting though not uncontroversial research into early child language.

Studying Syntactic Development

Much of what we know about the development of syntax comes, of course, from studying what children actually say. Longitudinal studies of children in their homes, talking with their mothers or fathers, have produced vast quantities of raw data in the form of transcripts. In order to find out what the child knows of syntactic rules at any given stage, the researcher must examine the full corpus of speech, looking for patterns and regularities, searching through what is said for what is left unspoken, and contrasting the language at this stage with what came earlier and what will come later. These studies of spontaneous speech can tell us a great deal about the language produced by the child, but they do not reveal much about what the child can or cannot understand. Nor do they tell us what the child might have been able to say but was never given the opportunity to do so. Because of these limitations, spontaneous speech data need to be complemented with more controlled, experimental studies that are designed to test children's comprehension of various syntactic forms, or their ability to produce or judge particular constructions in less natural but more controlled situations.

In this chapter we utilize both sources of evidence—spontaneous speech and controlled experiments—in describing the course of syntactic development. However, we depend more on spontaneous speech, which has been most widely used by researchers studying a variety of languages and provides us with the least problematic source of child language data since it is elicited in naturalistic contexts.

Entering the Complex Linguistic System

One of the most difficult issues about acquiring language that the child faces is how to break into the system. How do children manage to break up the steady stream of sounds they hear into basic units like words and morphemes? How do they learn to map specific sound sequences onto meanings? And how do they learn to figure out the basic grammatical categories of their language such as nouns, verbs, and adjectives? These are some of the fundamental questions about language acquisition that child language researchers must also address in their theories, even though young children at the earliest stages of development provide us with few clues.

One interesting hypothesis that has received some empirical support has been suggested by Morgan (1986), among others. According to Morgan, if adults were providing information in their speech to children about where boundaries exist, not only between words but also between phrases, the task of acquiring language would become feasible and simplified.

There does appear to be evidence that mothers and fathers provide strong intonational evidence about word and phrase boundaries, not only in English, but also in other languages, such as French and Japanese (Fernald et al., 1989). More importantly, there is also evidence that infants are sensitive to the salience of the information sent in pauses (Kemler Nelson, Hirsh-Pasek, Jusczyk, & Cassidy, 1989).

Once the child has broken the stream of speech into words, he may use other "bootstraps" into the syntactic system. Some researchers have suggested that meaning, or *semantics,* plays a key bootstrapping role for the child (e.g., Pinker, 1984); others suggest that the functions of language, or *pragmatics,* provide the primary route into the abstract grammatical system (e.g., Bates & MacWhinney, 1982). A third alternative is that grammar provides its own bootstrapping operation, suggesting that it operates as an independent cognitive system. We will consider the role that semantics, pragmatics, and grammar play in facilitating grammatical development at each of the different stages of the process.

Measuring Syntactic Growth

As children get older, their sentences grow longer. Recent studies of large numbers of children have provided excellent normative data on the age at which English-speaking children make the transition to combining words and using simple sentences. These data come from a set of parental report measures called the *Communicative Development Inventories* (Fenson, Dale, Reznick, Thal, Bates, Hartung, Pethick & Reilly, 1993; Fenson, Dale, Reznick, Bates, Thal, & Pethick, 1994), which provide highly reliable information about children's language abilities at the early stages. There is wide variability in the onset of combinatorial language. Some children begin as early as fifteen months, the average seems to be at about eighteen months, and by the age of two almost all children are producing some word combinations (Bates, Dale, & Thal, 1995). While age itself is not a good predictor of language development since children develop at vastly different rates, the length of a child's sentences is an excellent indicator of syntactic development; each new element of syntactic knowledge adds length to a child's utterances. Roger Brown (1973) introduced the major measure of syntactic development, the **mean length of utterance** or **MLU,** which is based on the average length of a child's sentences scored on transcripts of spontaneous speech. Length is determined by the number of meaningful units, or *morphemes,* rather than words. Morphemes include simple content words such as *cat, play, do, red;* function words such as *no, the, you, this;* and affixes or grammatical inflections such as *un-, -s, -ed.* The addition of each morpheme (or minimal unit carrying meaning) reflects the acquisition of new linguistic knowledge. So children who have similar MLUs are at the same level of linguistic maturity, and their language is at the same level of complexity.

In order to calculate the MLU of a particular child, one needs a transcript of a half-hour conversation. The child's language must be divided into separate utterances, and these utterances must be divided into morphemes. Brown (1973) provides detailed rules for judging what constitutes a morpheme for the child learning English (see Figure 5.4). For example, although compound words like *birthday* or *goodnight* contain two morphemes, they only count as one. The same is true for diminutives (e.g., *doggie, ducky*) and irregular past tense verbs (e.g., *got, did*). On the other hand, inflections (e.g., regular past tense *-ed,* plural *-s,* progressive *-ing*) and auxiliaries (e.g., *is, have, will*) count as separate morphemes. The number of morphemes in each of the first 100 fully transcribed utterances is counted, and the total is then divided by 100 (see Figure 5.4).

1. Start with the second page of the transcription unless that page involves a recitation of some kind. In this latter case, start with the first recitation-free stretch. Count the first 100 utterances satisfying the following rules.

2. Only fully transcribed utterances are used; none with blanks. Portions of utterances, entered in parentheses to indicate doubtful transcription, are used.

3. Include all exact utterance repetitions (marked with a plus sign in records). Stuttering is marked as repeated efforts at a single word; count the word once in the most complete form produced. In the few cases where a word is produced for emphasis or the like (*no, no, no*) count each occurrence.

4. Do not count such fillers as *mm* or *oh*, but do count *no, yeah,* and *hi*.

5. All compound words (two or more free morphemes), proper names, and ritualized reduplications count as single words. Examples: *birthday, rackety-boom, choo-choo, quack-quack, night-night, pocketbook, see saw.* Justification is that no evidence that the constituent morphemes function as such for these children.

6. Count as one morpheme all irregular pasts of the verb (*got, did, went, saw*). Justification is that there is no evidence that the child relates these to present forms.

7. Count as one morpheme all diminutives (*doggie, mommie*) because these children at least do not seem to use the suffix productively. Diminutives are the standard forms used by the child.

8. Count as separate morphemes all auxiliaries (*is, have, will, can, must, would*). Also all catenatives: *gonna, wanna, hafta.* These latter counted as single morphemes rather than as *going to* or *want to* because evidence is that they function so for the children. Count as separate morphemes all inflections, for example, possessive {s}, plural {s}, third person singular {s}, regular past {d}, progressive {in}.

9. The range count follows the above rules but is always calculated for the total transcription rather than for 100 utterances.

Figure 5.4

Rules for calculating mean length of utterance (Reprinted by permission of the publishers from *A First Language* by Roger Brown, Cambridge, MA: Harvard University Press, Copyright 1973 by the President and Fellows of Harvard College.)

In longitudinal studies, the MLUs calculated at successive points in time gradually increase. Figure 5.5 shows the MLU plotted against chronological age for the three children studied by Brown and his colleagues. Clearly, MLU grows at different rates in different children. Of the children followed by Brown, Eve's MLU rose most sharply, indicating very rapid language development, whereas Sarah and Adam showed more gradual and less consistent increments in their MLU. According to the MLU norms developed by Miller and Chapman (1981), based on a sample of over 100 middle-class children in Madison, Wisconsin (see Figure 5.6), Adam and Sarah are about average for their age, whereas Eve is very much advanced for her age. Using the MLU, Brown subdivided the major period of syntactic growth into five stages,

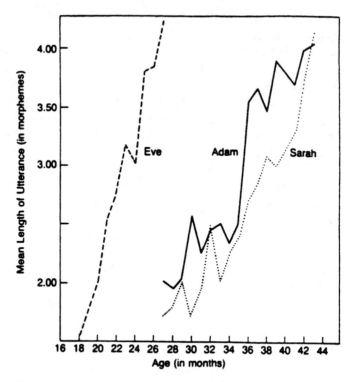

Figure 5.5

Mean length of utterance and chronological age of three children
(Reprinted by permission of the publishers from *A First Language* by R.
Brown, Cambridge, MA: Harvard University Press. Copyright 1973 by the
President and Fellows of Harvard College.)

beginning with Stage I when the MLU is between 1.0 and 2.0. Successive stages are
marked by increments of .5; thus, Stage II goes from 2.0 to 2.5, Stage III is from 2.5
to 3.0, Stage IV is from 3.0 to 3.5, and Stage V is from 3.5 to 4.0. Beyond an MLU
of about 4.0 some of the assumptions on which the measure is based are no longer
valid, and longer sentences do not simply reflect what the child knows about language; so MLU loses value as an index of language development after this stage.

There are some questions that arise in calculating MLUs (e.g., should one
include yes/no responses to adult questions?), and these have led to some criticisms of
it as an index of syntactic development (Crystal, 1974). Nevertheless, it has proven
immensely useful as a means of classifying children in the early stages of syntactic
development, and it remains an important tool for research and clinical assessment of
English-speaking children. More serious problems are encountered in measuring the
MLU in foreign languages, especially highly inflected and synthetic languages such as
German, Russian, or Hebrew. In these cases it becomes difficult to decide what func-

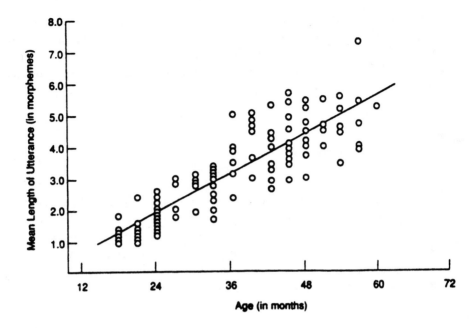

Figure 5.6

Source: From "The Relations between Age and Mean Length of Utterance" by J. F. Miller and R. S. Chapman, 1981, *Journal of Speech and Hearing Research, 24*, pp. 154–161.

tions as a morpheme in the child's speech, and it is easy to obtain inflated numbers. Still, there have been attempts to extend the concept of MLU to structurally varied languages (Bowerman, 1973) or to modify the measure to account for cross-linguistic differences (Dromi & Berman, 1982). In some languages calculating the length of utterances in words, rather than morphemes has proven to be quite useful. One example comes from a recent study on the acquisition of Irish (Hickey, 1991). It remains to be seen how well this or some other related measure would apply to other languages. By using a similar index to chart language growth across a range of languages, we can search for the universal and invariant features that characterize the main stages of syntactic development.

Recently, there have been advances made in developing additional measures of syntactic development. One example is the **Index of Productive Syntax,** or **IPSyn,** introduced by Hollis Scarborough (1989). For this measure one also needs a transcript of 100 spontaneous speech utterances from a child. Using the scoresheet provided by Scarborough, the researcher marks the use, up to a maximum of two very different uses, of a variety of structures in four categories: in noun phrases (e.g., nouns, pronouns, articles, plural endings, compound nouns), verb phrases (verbs, prepositions, verb endings, auxiliaries, modals, tense), questions and negation forms (at various levels of complexity), and sentence structure (simple, complex, complements, conjunctions, infinitive forms). The score received is simply the total number of points, with points awarded for each structure used. The IPSyn measure correlates very highly with MLU, demonstrating its validity as a measure of grammatical development. However, it has the advantage of providing a measure that remains useful far beyond the MLU limit of 4.0, at least until around five years of age.

Two-Word Utterances

The first stage defined by Brown follows children through their earliest attempts at multiword utterances, as the MLU grows from 1.0 to 2.0. Most of the child's sentences are two words long, although a few may be as long as three or even four words. Table 5.1 lists numerous examples of two-word sentences taken from separate children acquiring English as their first language. Examples from children learning other languages are very similar to these.

Table 5.1 **Examples of Two-Word Utterances**

Andrew	*Eve*
more car	bye-bye baby
more cereal	Daddy bear
more high	Daddy book
more read	Daddy honey
outside more	there Daddy
no more	there potty
no pee	more pudding
no wet	Mommy stair
all wet	Mommy dimple
all gone	Mommy do
bye-bye Calico	Mommy bear
bye-bye back	eat it
bye-bye car	read it
bye-bye Papa	see boy
Mama come	more cookie
see pretty	

Note: Terms in column 1 are from Braine, 1976; those in column 2 are from Eve's transcripts and from Brown and Fraser, 1963.

Looking at these examples, we can note a number of interesting features about children's early sentences. First, from the beginning the child's language is truly creative; many of these sentences would never have been spoken by an adult. The particular word combinations spoken by Stage I children are unique and novel rather than mere imitations of adult sentences. Second, these sentences are simple, compared to adult sentences, and simplicity is accomplished in a systematic way. Certain words called *content* or **open-class** words dominate the children's language. Thus, their sentences are composed primarily of nouns, verbs, and adjectives. These large word classes are called open since they freely admit new items and drop old ones as a language evolves. In contrast, *function words* or **closed-class words** are usually missing at this stage of language development. The closed word classes (including prepositions, conjunctions, articles, pronouns, auxiliaries, and inflections) are much smaller and do not change their composition readily. The absence of these grammatical terms lends to the impression of simplicity. We can also notice that some words are very frequent in a particular child's corpus (Andrew uses *more* and *bye-bye* often and in combination with many different words), and the order of the words appears quite regular. Finally, if we look at what the children are talking about, we can see that certain topics (such as possession, location, recurrence) are very prevalent.

Investigators of child language have spent the last twenty years trying to come up with the best, most accurate way of characterizing Stage I language. There have been a number of changes in these characterizations as the focus shifted from one significant feature to another. However, these changes do not reflect differences in the data but in the kinds of categories imposed on the data by different researchers. The challenge is to ascribe neither too little nor too much knowledge of syntactic categories or rules to the child just beginning to acquire syntax.

Telegraphic Speech

The earliest characterizations of Stage I language focused on the contrast between the open-class and closed-class words. Brown and Fraser (1963) called these two-word utterances **telegraphic** because the omission of closed-class words makes them resemble telegrams. In fact, not all of the words used are from the open classes. A small handful of functors like *more, no, you,* and *off* are scattered throughout the transcripts and can be seen in the examples in Table 5.1. Miller and Ervin (1964) suggested that children choose just those words that are highly stressed in adult language and are thus perceptually more salient. These include nouns, adjectives, and verbs and also some closed-class words, especially those that are syllabic and express semantic information (Brown, 1973). Gleitman and Wanner (1982) have suggested that children, in fact, learn open- and closed-class words quite separately. The earlier acquisition of open-class words is based on their perceptual salience, according to Gleitman and Wanner, and thus represents a good example of prosodic features helping the child to discover basic language structure.

The idea that Stage I language consists exclusively of open-class words comes from research on the acquisition of English. More recent studies that have looked at children acquiring other languages, for example, Italian (Hyams, 1986a, 1989), Turkish (Aksu-Koc, 1988), or Hebrew (Levy, 1988), which have much richer morphological systems and may be less reliant on words to express basic grammatical relations, have shown that even at the earliest stages children acquiring these kinds of languages are also beginning to acquire some of the closed-class morphology.

Semantic Relations

Studies of children from around the world in Stage I, using two-word utterances, have shown that one universal feature of this stage is that only a small group of meanings, or **semantic relations**, is expressed in the children's language. Bloom (1970) first observed this in her study of three American children. Later, Brown (1973) extended her findings to children acquiring Finnish, Swedish, Samoan, Spanish, French, Russian, Korean, Japanese, and Hebrew. Table 5.2 lists the eight most prevalent combinatorial meanings found by Brown (pp. 193–197) along with some examples of each.

From these examples we see that during Stage I children talk a great deal about objects—they point them out and name them (demonstrative) and they talk about where the objects are (location), what they are like (attributive), who owns them (possession), and who is doing things to them (agent-object). They also talk about actions performed by people (agent-action), performed on objects (action-object), and oriented toward certain locations (action-location). Objects, people, and actions and their interrelationships thus preoccupy the toddler universally, and, as Brown points out, these are precisely the concepts that the child has just completed differentiating during what Piaget has called the sensorimotor stage of cognitive development.

Table 5.2 Set of Prevalent Semantic Relations in Stage I

Semantic Relation	*Examples*
agent + action	mommy come; daddy sit
action + object	drive car; eat grape
agent + object	mommy sock; baby book
action + location	go park; sit chair
entity + location	cup table; toy floor
possessor + possession	my teddy; mommy dress
entity + attribute	box shiny; crayon big
demonstrative + entity	dat money; dis telephone

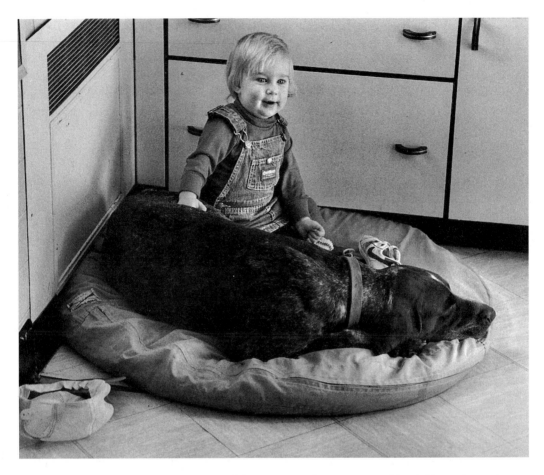

"My doggie." Possessor + possession is one of the semantic relations expressed by children who are just beginning to combine 2 words into Stage I speech.

Early Grammar

Another important feature of children's two-word utterances is their consistent word order. In his study, Brown (1973) used the children's correct use of word order as evidence in support of the semantic relations approach to Stage I. Braine (1963, 1976) also has documented the early productive use of word order rules for children acquiring a variety of languages. He noted, however, that early two-word combinations had more limited, lexical-specific scope than either Bloom or Brown had suggested, which he called **limited scope formulae**. Moreover, Braine (1976) showed that there were large individual differences in the order in which different semantic relations were acquired.

Pinker (1984, 1987) has taken the findings about Stage I speech to argue that children use semantics to provide the key bootstrap into the linguistic system. The child can use the correspondence between things and names to map onto the linguistic category of nouns. Names for physical attributes or changes of state are expressed as verbs. Because all sentence subjects at this stage are essentially semantic agents, children can use this syntactic-semantic correspondence to begin figuring out the abstract syntactic relations for more complex sentences that require the category of subject, but which are not clearly agents too.

Paul Bloom (1990a) provides some interesting evidence for this general idea that semantics may bootstrap the child directly into the grammatical system. He found that from the start children assign words to syntactic categories such as noun, verb, and adjective. Even in Stage I, children learning English know that pronouns and proper nouns are different from common nouns because adjectives can only come before the latter. Thus the first sentence below is grammatical, but the other sentences (marked with an *) are not:

The *big dog* runs away.
*Small *she* goes home.
*Happy Fred is here.

Looking through the transcripts from children in Stage I, Bloom found that children almost never violated this word order rule of English, and seemed therefore to know the difference between common nouns, pronouns, and proper nouns. At the same time, Gleitman (1990) argues that very young children also seem able to use syntax to provide them clues about semantics or the meanings of words, and there is some evidence for this hypothesis (Naigles, 1990).

How does the evidence about very early child language fit in with the linguistic theory proposed in GB theory? One answer to this question comes from a British linguist, Andrew Radford (1990), who argues that much of the linguistic system is absent in Stage I, but what the child does have at this stage is a lexicon and a limited set of phrase structure rules in d-structure. Specifically, Radford claims that English-speaking children at Stage I only have lexical categories; what is missing from their grammars are the functional categories such as INFL and COMP. There is also no transformational rule; however, the d-structure does get assigned thematic roles to yield the s-structure. These ideas are very similar to the other descriptions of Stage I language that we have discussed earlier, but Radford uses the terminology and framework of the GB theory.

Another use of the GB framework to explain Stage I grammar has been proposed by Hyams (1986a, 1989). If one looks at the examples of Stage I utterances listed in Table 5.1 that contain verbs (e.g., *eat it*), one notices that these utterances lack a subject. Hyams suggests that this is the result of the **null-subject parameter,** which starts off in all children in the position for languages, like Italian, that allow subjectless sentences. According to Hyams, all children begin with the parameter set one way (e.g., the Italian way), and so English-speaking children eventually have to switch the setting of the parameter to the other position. During Stage I, when English-speaking children often omit subjects and do not have any expletive pronouns in their language, their grammars conform to this setting.

Although Hyams's hypothesis is attractive because it is theoretically grounded, there have been some important criticisms raised by other researchers (O'Grady, Peters, & Masterson, 1989). Valian (1990) points out some logical problems with the claim that parameters start off in one particular setting. She also provides evidence that even though American children at the early stages of language development omit subjects, they do, in fact, include a sentence subject significantly more often than do Italian children at the same stage of development, suggesting that they know that subjects need to be expressed. But if they know that subjects must be included in a sentence, why do young children omit them frequently? Bloom (1990b) shows that the problem for young children is that they have a limited processing capacity—they can only cope with producing utterances of limited length, and this constrains which elements will be included in a sentence and which will be omitted. Subjects are omitted more frequently than objects (which are also occasionally absent) either because of processing limitations (since subjects come at the beginning of a sentence and this places a heavier processing load than do elements, like objects, which appear at ends of sentences) or for pragmatic reasons (the subject of a sentence is often provided by context, or has been established in prior discourse). Finally, Ingham (1992) reports a recent case study which found that the acquisition of obligatory sentence subjects in English was not tied to other developments in the child's grammar, as would be predicted on Hyam's theory.

Controversies about the nature of children's early grammars, the role of GB theory, and the best way to conceptualize the child's early linguistic system have yet to be resolved. This extensive look at one stage in the acquisition of grammar highlights the importance of both theories in motivating new research and a closer, more detailed look at children's language, for English as well as other languages.

Children's Early Comprehension of Syntax

Thus far we have presented a picture of early language development that is based entirely on studies of spontaneous speech production. These studies, however, leave unanswered a host of questions about young children's comprehension of syntax. We might ask, for example, when children begin to comprehend two or more word utterances. Is comprehension in advance of production or *vice versa*? What is the relationship between comprehension and production?

Parents generally believe that their children are understanding multiword utterances almost from the time they begin using their first words, and that comprehension is clearly in advance of production. Unfortunately, until very recently, research on this issue yielded conflicting results. For example, some studies supported the parents' view that children understand more than they can say (e.g., Fraser, Bellugi, & Brown, 1963; Huttenlocher, 1974; Sachs & Truswell, 1978), while others found that children could say more than they really understood (e.g., Chapman, 1977) or that the two abilities were at about the same level (e.g., Roberts, 1983). Of course, one difficulty in comparing different studies is that researchers have used very different methods for assessing comprehension while ensuring that children could not be relying on context to interpret the linguistic message (cf. Leonard, 1983). Different methods that have been used to assess comprehension include diary studies (which document conditions under which the child can or cannot understand); act-out tasks (in which the experimenter asks the child to act out a sentence using toys—e.g., "Make the girl kiss the duck"); direction tasks (in which the child is asked to carry out a direction, such as "Tickle the duck"); and picture-choice tasks (in which the child must select the picture that best represents the linguistic form being tested). There are serious limitations with each of these methods that have led to the confusion in the literature regarding children's comprehension abilities.

In recent years, Golinkoff and Hirsh-Pasek have pioneered the use of the **preferential looking paradigm** for assessing language comprehension in infants as young as twelve months old, which avoids all the problems of other techniques. Using this new method, these researchers have found that even in the single-word stage, seventeen-month-old children can use word order to comprehend multiword utterances (Golinkoff & Hirsh-Pasek, 1987; Golinkoff, Hirsh-Pasek, Cauley, & Gordon, 1987). Their method (illustrated in Figure 5.7) involves setting the child on its mother's lap equidistant from two video monitors. While the mother closes her eyes and makes no attempt to communicate with her child, the child watches two simultaneously presented color videos. The linguistic message, presented over a centrally placed loudspeaker in synchrony with the videotaped scenes, directs the child to attend to one of the monitors. A hidden experimenter directly observes the child's eye movements and records the amount of time spent watching the two videos on each trial.

Hirsh-Pasek and Golinkoff (1993) have used this paradigm to assess comprehension of various language features. For example, one key comparison they used to test comprehension of word order involved observing very young children while they heard the sentence "Cookie Monster is tickling Big Bird." One of the video scenes had Cookie Monster tickling Big Bird, while in the other scene, simultaneously presented, Big Bird was tickling Cookie Monster. Because children at seventeen months of age reliably spent longer looking at the former scene, Golinkoff and Hirsh-Pasek (1995) concluded that children can comprehend word order before they even begin using two-word sentences.

These findings suggest that comprehension is indeed in advance of production, as parents have always known. Children are thus able to exploit knowledge gained from listening to adult speech to guide the acquisition of grammatical forms. Future

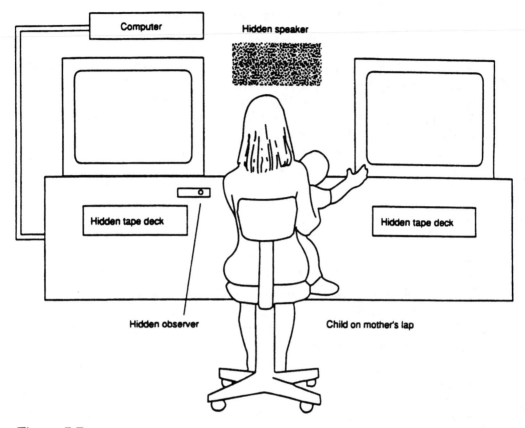

Figure 5.7

Experimental setup of the preferential looking paradigm (From Naigles, 1990)

studies perhaps will tell us whether comprehension development follows the same stages that have been found in the development of spontaneous speech.

Developing Grammatical Morphemes

When we look at children's language as it develops beyond Stage I, we notice two important changes. One is that sentences get longer as children begin combining two or more basic semantic relations. For example, agent + action and action + object may be combined to yield agent + action + object, as in "Adam hit ball." In this way sentences also become progressively more complex in content. The second change is the gradual appearance of a few inflections and other closed-class terms that, "like an intricate sort of ivy, begin to grow up between and upon the major construction blocks, the nouns and verbs, to which Stage I is largely limited" (Brown, 1973, p. 249).

The process of acquiring the major *grammatical morphemes* is gradual and lengthy. Some are still not fully controlled until the child enters school (for example, certain irregular past-tense verbs). Nevertheless, the process begins early, as soon as the MLU approaches 2.0, and we will discuss the main research findings on the acquisition of a small subset of fourteen English grammatical morphemes.

The development of these morphemes was studied by Brown and his colleague Courtney Cazden (1968) using the longitudinal data from Adam, Eve, and Sarah (Brown, 1973). The fourteen morphemes were selected both because they were very frequent and because one can easily identify the contexts in which they are needed to produce a grammatically well-formed sentence.

The Fourteen Morphemes

Grammatical morphemes, even though they do not carry independent meaning, do subtly shade the meaning of sentences. The morpheme group studied by Brown included two prepositions (*in, on*), two articles (*a, the*), noun inflections marking possessive (*'s*) and plural (*-s*), verb inflections marking progressive (*-ing*), third-person present tense of regular verbs (e.g., he walk*s*) or irregular verbs (e.g., he *has*), past tense of regular verbs (e.g., he walk*ed*) and irregular verbs (e.g., *had*), and the main uses of the verb *to be*—as auxiliary, both when it can be contracted (e.g., I *am* walking or I'*m* walking) and when it cannot be contracted (e.g., I *was* walking), and as a main verb or *copula* in its contractible form (e.g., I *am* happy or I'*m* happy) and its uncontractible form (e.g., This *is* it).

In order to chart the development of these morphemes, Brown closely examined each child utterance to identify whether it required any of the morphemes to make it fully grammatical by adult standards. Both the linguistic context (the utterance itself) and the nonlinguistic context can be used to decide which morphemes are necessary. For example, when a child says "that book" while pointing out a book, we know that there should be a copula (*'s* or *is*) and an article (*a*). Or if a child says "two book table" when there are a couple of books lying on the table, we know that *book* should have a plural *-s* and the preposition *on* and article *the* are required before the word *table*. In this way Brown went through the transcripts of his three subjects from Stage I to Stage V and identified all of the obligatory contexts for each morpheme. Then he checked how many of these contexts were actually filled with the appropriate morphemes at the different stages of development. From this he calculated the percentage of each morpheme actually supplied in its obligatory context for each child for each sample of spontaneous speech. This measure has the advantage of being independent of actual frequency of use since frequency may vary considerably from one child to another and from one point in time to the next.